James Rogers worked as a child psychiatrist for over four decades. He qualified from the London Hospital in 1941 and, after four three-month training jobs, he joined the Royal Navy. His first ship, a destroyer, was sunk in the Mediterranean in September 1943. After five months, he joined another ship which went to the Normandy beaches on D Day. Two days later she was sunk and James received multiple injuries. He was invalided from the navy in 1946. He then did five years post-graduate work, obtaining the MRCP and DPM. He then went to the Crichton Royal Hospital in Dumfries, where he helped to set up and run the pioneering Ladyfield children's unit. He then went to the Royal Hospital for Sick Children in Edinburgh, where he was also a Senior Lecturer at the University. Here he extended his work to include schools, children's homes and foster homes. Since retiring he has moved to Rockcliffe, an estuary on the Solway.

METAMORPHOSES

Troubled Children Over Four Decades

James Rogers

Book Guild Publishing
Sussex, England

First published in Great Britain in 2009 by
The Book Guild
Pavilion View
19 New Road
Brighton, BN1 1UF

Typesetting in Times by
Keyboard Services, Luton, Bedfordshire

Printed in Great Britain by
Athenaeum Press Ltd, Gateshead

A catalogue record for this book is available from
The British Library

ISBN 978 1 84624 354 7

CONTENTS

INTRODUCTION

This book is an account of some of the changes that have taken place in the field of child psychiatry over four decades. It is also an account of some remarkable changes that have taken place in some very disturbed children.

Part 1 is about the work of an experienced psychiatrist in a hospital setting with adequate resources and a dedicated and skilled staff. This is a very expensive provision even though, as in the case of Ladyfield, the salaries of the teachers and the school equipment were paid by the Local Authority. The setting was the Department of Child Psychiatry at the Crichton Royal Hospital in Dumfries, and the time was the early 1950s. The children's unit was in a pleasant house in its own grounds outside the grounds of the main hospital. There were 20 children, and later another two houses each in its own grounds were added to the Children's Department, but at first I had the one house. The care staff were nurses recruited from the hospital, men and women. A small core had both general and psychiatric training. The rest were what was called State Enrolled Nurses. They had all had training. In the rest of the hospital there were always nurses under training who moved about among the different units. I managed to establish that Ladyfield, the children's unit, had its staff appointed specifically to it. Any staff under training could only come as supernumeraries. I recognised the importance of the children being able to form lasting relationships with the staff and this they did. The staff also included an educational psychologist, a teacher and an occupational therapist. I was initially the only doctor. Consultants usually had senior registrars, registrars and house physicians. At first I had none of these. Later when the department grew I had all of these, but at first I had none, so I did everything. If a child fell out of a tree I patched him or her up. If they had a sore throat I peered down it. If they broke several windows at 3 a.m. I stalked across a field and acted the heavy father. I think I always realised how lucky I was. I formed a very close relationship with the staff; I was entirely dependent on them and they were entirely dependent on me.

Part 2 describes the work of a psychiatrist in a hospital setting but with his work in an advisory capacity extended to a large number of institutions: children's homes, schools and organisations providing foster parents.

Part 3 describes the practical work of a psychiatrist, not hospital based, in schools, and it could be in children's homes and with foster homes. This work could also be done by a psychologist, a social worker or a teacher provided they had the relevant skill and experience. There are a large number of schools who cater for children who have failed in mainstream schools. There are hundreds of teachers in those schools and thousands of children attending them. The need for this type of help is great.

I will now talk about some of the children and then look at how the changes may have taken place.

Part 1

Ladyfield

CHAPTER 1

Iris

Iris was referred to my unit when she was eight years old. She was described as being difficult at home to the point of being impossible to live within the family. She wet the bed, soiled herself, had a poor appetite and walked with a limp though no physical abnormality had been found. Everything the family said about her was negative. She was the middle of three daughters, and she had been born when her father had been overseas for more than a year. Her father was a regular in the armed forces. Although Iris was clearly not his child he accepted her as a member of the family and he and his wife then had another daughter. In spite of having been accepted as a member of the family Iris was always the 'odd one out'. For example, when the children had to have new winter coats, Iris had the one passed on from the older child. This seems a trivial example but it was typical of a great many ways in which Iris was made to feel she was a second-class citizen. The fact was that both her sisters had new coats and she had the passed-down one. This was typical of Iris's experiences.

When Iris came to the residential unit she was just as negative as she had been described by the family. She was listless, uninterested, timid and altogether unchildlike. I started seeing her for therapy sessions, at first four times weekly. To begin with the sessions were rather dreary. She did not seem interested in the toys, the sand tray or anything else. Nor did she want to talk. After a few weeks she began to play more. She arranged the animals in the sand tray and talked about them. She put the mothers with the children in one field but always put the fathers in another field some way away from the rest of the family. She remarked: 'Fathers never have much to do with children do they?'

Parents were encouraged to visit the children regularly. The children normally went home for holidays and all other forms of contact – letters, phone calls and parcels were encouraged and recorded. Iris was left in total isolation. The social worker wrote and visited the family and I wrote. There was always some excuse: the car would not start, someone was ill, etc. Iris was encouraged to write and she did frequently. When she wrote letters with me I sent them unedited, with blots, spelling mistakes – a mess, but a heart-rending mess. When the letters were finished Iris and I would go outside to a postbox, and when I had put a stamp on, Iris would carefully post them.

Iris was still very timid. The children always went swimming twice a week and for most this was one of the highlights of the week, but Iris used to plead to have her session with me at the swimming time, with which I agreed. She began painting. At first her pictures were all of isolated places where there were no people and nothing ever happened. The stage of *Waiting for Godot* would have been a cheerful place compared to the bleak landscapes Iris took me to. At least the two tramps had each other to talk to, but Iris's places were totally bleak. Later she painted a picture of a place with bars on the windows where all the nice people were shut up. The only way out was through a maze, and the only people who could get you through the maze were the witches, but when they got to the end of the maze they usually ate you. I thought the bad place was the unit where Iris was living. Needless to say there were no bars on the windows nor were the doors locked except at night. I thought I was one of the witches – one of those clever people who pretended to help you but who were in fact dangerous. I did not at this stage interpret any of this to Iris.

Iris went back to the sand tray. I suggested we made a circus. Iris immediately changed the game. She said, 'We won't have a circus, we will have Cinderella.' So we made a carriage and Iris arranged two people, the prince and princess in the carriage and then put Cinderella in the carriage with them. I had previously introduced Iris's two sisters and Iris had put them on the other side of the fence. I said to Iris, 'You would like to be Cinderella wouldn't you (close to mother and father with the sisters on the other side of the fence)?' She agreed but I did not carry this any further.

A few days later I was in the unit at about 8 p.m. I heard some sobbing coming from the girls' bedroom. This was an unusual sound in the unit. Not that children did not cry but when they did they usually had gained a good deal of security and were as much angry as sad. This was a very sad 'head under the bedclothes' kind of crying so I went to investigate. Iris said someone had hit her. I said I did not think that would cause so much grief. Iris said she was not going to tell me anyway, and she did not want to see me. I stayed and eventually she came down to my room. There she said, 'I'm crying because I am never going to have a happy life – my mummy does not want me, my daddy does not want me and if your mummy and daddy don't want you no one is going to want you and you will not have a happy life.' All of which was true but not easy to face up to at that age or indeed at any age. I said to her that at present the situation at home was a very unhappy one but I had seen families where things were as bad but there had been a happy ending. Iris did not think this was likely in her case and nor did I. So I suggested to her that if things didn't work out with the family could her happiness come from outside the family? And I reminded her about Cinderella whom she had introduced

5

into the play a few days ago. She said that might be so but nobody liked her. I asked if anyone liked her. She said she thought I liked her or I would not see her so often. I assured her that I really did like her, but was there anyone else who liked her? She said she thought the Sister liked her a bit. I then alerted Sister, head of the care staff to this. Sister was one of those amazing people who could make one child feel she was the apple of her eye without the other children noticing. In these cases the whole staff had to be aware of what was going on in therapy. This required a very high degree of trust by all staff. Sister gave the necessary encouragement and Iris used to ask to go to the toilet in school and disappear for 20 minutes or so while she went off for a good cuddle. The teacher who, like all staff, knew what was going on, made no comment.

At this time Iris began to improve markedly. She was much more confident and began to play happily with the other children. Then I heard that there was trouble in the girls' bedroom. There were two other girls in Iris's room, one older and one younger, very much matching the family pattern. We heard that the two younger girls had ganged up and were giving the older one a bad time. I suggested to the staff that they did not try to resolve this but to give the older girl a lot of fuss to make her feel better. Then we heard that Iris had changed sides and the two older girls were giving the younger one a bad time. I translated this to her home life and I asked Iris what it felt like to have – I named her younger sister here – under her thumb. Iris grinned and said it felt great. This soon settled down and they were all good friends again. Iris then went through a phase of being awkward with members of the staff. With the teacher she had been biddable though not doing much work. Now she became entirely negative and even abusive. She was equally awkward with the occupational therapist with whom she did group therapy. She used to complain that the therapist never seemed to have left-handed hammers. These phases were short-lived and soon she was functioning well in all fields and producing much better work and play. Her confidence had increased and she now enjoyed swimming. She would say to me sometimes, 'I don't want to see you this week.' But quite often she would suddenly demand to see me.

At this time we lost contact with the family altogether. The father was serving abroad and we could make no contact with the mother by letter or telephone. Then I had a phone call from the mother from the south of England (they had been living in Scotland), asking me to put the child on a plane at the nearest airport and she would meet her at Heathrow. This was clearly impossible in view of her mother's lack of any real concern for the child: we could not be certain she would meet the plane. She gave me an address and as in the near future I was going to a conference in that direction I said I would take the child with me to that address. I did this and when I went to the address the mother greeted Iris effusively. 'Come in, darling, this is your new daddy and here are your new brother and sister.' It transpired that the mother was living with a colleague of the father's by whom she had had twins. I left Iris with many misgivings. A few weeks later I was again in that part of the world so I went to the house to see how they were getting on. The woman who owned the house was rather suspicious at first but when I explained that I was the doctor who had brought the little girl she took me in and told me the story. The father had heard of the situation. He had got compassionate leave and come to the UK. He had dispatched the babies to a home to be put up for adoption and taken his original family, including Iris, abroad with him. The wife's partner shot himself.

I heard no more of Iris for a few years. Then I received a letter from a service base in the south of England asking for information about Iris, who was then about 14. I sent

JAMES ROGERS

very full reports and asked most earnestly for information from them. This did not come.

I next heard about Iris from a woman I had worked with at the Maudsley. She had married and was running a residential establishment for teenage girls. I had quite a bit of correspondence with her. The family had split up but Iris was doing well. This was an exceptional woman could give children a wonderful sense of security. Iris had become interested in breeding dogs.

I did not hear about Iris again for several years. Then one day a car drew up in front of my unit and out got a pretty girl with a baby on her arm and a dog. There was also a husband who seemed to be a very nice young man. This was Iris.

I have introduced the children at this early stage because their problems and the way we set about trying to help them is what this is all about. In psychiatry at this time there was great confusion about which theoretical models were relevant or even true. Some say the position is not so different now. So I will say a little more about how the unit ran and how the children were helped. First of all there was complete trust among the members of staff. From the beginning I emphasised that not only was it important that no information about the children was disclosed outside the unit but also that no one outside the unit knew about the children. Other people should not know that the staff were looking after children. This sounds a tall order but the children and I were never let down. Meetings of the whole staff took place each week and had I frequent talks with them in between. Everything about the children was shared including details of their individual therapy. With the degree of confidentiality we had established this was possible.

In Iris's case I think the therapy she had with me was important. In her play she told me that she was alone, unloved and unwanted. She was then able to say this plainly in words.

8

I suggested to her that perhaps, like Cinderella, she might find happiness outside the family. She did not think so but she took the hint. This was when she began asking to go out of school, presumably to go to the toilet. In fact she rushed upstairs to Sister and had a good cuddle lasting 20 minutes or more. Her idea of herself changed dramatically. She now saw herself as a loving and lovable person. She demanded and received affection from other members of staff. It was then that she started her little awkward phases, with the teacher and with the occupational therapist. Having found out that she was as much loved then as ever, she was able to abandon these awkward phases and continued as a cheerful, helpful and loving child. Although I did not see her again for many years, she managed somehow to retain this loving image of herself Perhaps her mother became loving towards her, possibly as a substitute for her lost twins. I think her father continued to reject her because she eventually had to leave the family. The woman running the adolescent home she went to was a very warm and caring person. Whatever happened during her adolescent years, Iris managed to hang on to the loving image she had found at Ladyfield and to marry and have a family – and to come back to Ladyfield to say 'thank you'.

Simon

Simon was referred to me from a place 300 miles from my unit. I would not normally undertake to see anyone from such a distance, but the referring agent, a particularly caring children's officer, was in some despair about him. He was eight years old and had killed another child by pushing him over a dockside into the sea. The other child unfortunately became entangled in part of the dock structure and was drowned. Simon was tested and found to be of an intellectual

9

level well below chronological age. He was sent to an institution for mentally handicapped children. A report from there designated Simon as a 'dangerous psychopath who should be locked up for life'. The children's officer was concerned that a child of that age should be written off in this way, but not surprisingly had difficulty in finding anyone who would take him on even for assessment. I took him on initially for assessment. Treatment would only be undertaken if the assessment seemed to warrant it. Arrangements were made for the family to visit Simon whenever they could, and their fares would be paid and accommodation provided in Dumfries. A senior member of the children's department staff undertook the therapy for the family, keeping a close liaison with a social worker in my unit. The progress of this therapy will be described later.

When Simon arrived at the unit he was rather small for his age, a slight, pale boy who was quiet and seemed apprehensive. In all other cases I told the staff full details about the children. They respected the confidence and did not let anyone know they knew such details. In this case I told only the senior member of the care staff that Simon had killed another child.

The family history was a troubled one. The father was an intelligent man who had been denied further education by serious illness in his mid-teens. He felt 'hard done by' and had a chip on his shoulder. He obtained a job in the security department of a big concern. In the meantime he got married and Simon was born. He seemed to be doing well in his job. He had coped successfully with a number of emergencies and was well thought of until it was discovered that he had created the emergencies in order to cope with them. He was charged and went to prison for two years. This was a shattering blow to Simon's mother. She became depressed and virtually rejected Simon. She felt a pariah in her own community and kept to herself. Simon was kept in the house. When the father came home his strong, outgoing personality reasserted itself. They had two more children who grew up normally. Simon, however, did not recover from the traumatic isolation he had experienced. When he went to school he had no idea about how to get on with other children and was at times very aggressive, to the extent that he was often kept in the classroom at playtimes. It was one day after school that he pushed the other child over the dock with the disastrous consequences. There was no indication he meant to kill the child, but that was what occurred.

Simon settled so well in the unit that long-term treatment was started. This involved four main approaches. He had individual therapy with a skilled woman therapist, one hour three times weekly with additional sessions if these were indicated. He had group therapy with one other child weekly. He had the day-to-day care of the very skilled care staff, and he attended school, in a very small class in the building in which he lived.

There were remarkable differences in his reactions and his progress in these four spheres. With the care staff he made steady though slow progress, passing the developmental stages he had clearly missed out on in a steady and reasonable way, consistent with learning social and developmental skills he had missed out on. In the unit, where there were always care staff around whatever the children were doing, there were no signs of aggressive behaviour. And the staff had no difficulties in coping with Simon.

In his individual sessions the story was a very different one, and had a dramatic quality, which never appeared in his social learning with other staff members. During the first few sessions he showed great concern for his therapist. Was it warm enough for her? Would she like the window open? He obviously wanted to be liked. Then after a good number of not particularly interesting or meaningful play sessions he went through a stage of violent aggression, verbal as well

11

as physical. This was so severe that the therapist, a strong and very competent person, was on occasions reduced to tears. Simon never showed this behaviour to any other member of staff He then became friendly and at times affectionate again, and began to act out his hidden anxieties. The therapy room was on the third floor of the building. Simon found a plastic baby doll. This he threw out of the window. He ran off down the stairs and ran back with the doll, saying anxiously to his therapist, 'It's all right, it's not hurt, is it? I've made it all right haven't I?' This play was repeated several times. The therapist had to reassure him many times that the doll was quite all right. There followed a further spell of friendly and fairly ordinary play, punctuated by several more aggressive sessions, though not as severe as the original one. On several occasions he was very affectionate and wanted to sit on the therapist's knee and have a lot of cuddling. He then enlisted the therapist's help in constructing a model in Plasticine, which was clearly a representation of the dock where the accident took place. This play was also repeated several times.

Eventually, after nine months of therapy, Simon was able to talk directly about the accident itself. His therapist asked him if he ever thought about the child who died. Simon said, 'I pray for him every night.' He was given a great deal of reassurance that the death really was an accident.

In the meantime work went on with the family. At first the social worker invited both parents to visit him in his office. They never seemed able to come. So he started home visits. The father was always out, or went out almost immediately the social worker arrived. The mother gained much from the visits and found that her views were valued. She gained greatly in confidence. The father saw how much she had gained and made a point of now being there when the social worker came so that he could monopolise the conversation. The mother felt hard done by and started making appointments to see the social worker in his office. They finished up having most of their sessions all together in the office, together with occasional home visits. Only by this time, the mother had gained enough confidence to make her full contribution to the discussions. The parents were encouraged to visit the unit. The mother did but the father did not.

Simon's steady progress continued until in all respects he was behaving as a normal boy. There were still problems at home in that the other children in the street were apt to tease him and bring up the incident. So it was decided he should go to a residential school for educationally limited children, the school being about 35 miles from home. We kept in close touch with the family and after a year heard that the family were unhappy about the school and there were several other problems. So the social worker from the unit who had done all the liaison work and I went to see them. We visited the school and found that Simon was top boy there and that the educational psychologist had recently found him to be functioning at a normal level in every field. Because of his early difficulties and the interruption to his schooling he still had some catching up to do. The parents had not been fully informed of his very good progress in school. I thought it was a bit harsh that I had to come down from Scotland to remedy failures in local communications. However, at the end of the visit we were delighted to see the family so well and happy.

There were a number of interesting aspects of this case. With the family, the mother's traumatic experience of her husband going to prison meant she was in no state to give Simon the care and affection he needed and he was ill-equipped to cope with the teasing he got from the other children when he emerged from the almost total isolation to which he had been subjected. He had no opportunity to learn the ordinary give and take of children's relationships. He was also inhibited in his cognitive development. By the time he came to the unit he was three to four years retarded in his cognitive as well as his emotional development. The family were unable to help him to free himself from the heavy burden of guilt he bore. The father had succeeded at least on the surface by putting all these traumatic experiences behind him. The mother on the other hand was haunted by these experiences, and it was not until she gained confidence as a result of her many talks with the social workers that she was able to play her full part in the family affairs. As she was a very warm and caring person and also had a great deal of common sense, this was of considerable importance.

In the course of time and with skilled help the dynamics of the family did change. The help came from the social worker in the unit as well as the one locally, who kept closely in touch with each other. Simon's handling by the care staff, an essential part of his therapy, enabled him to grow up and eventually reach his full potential. This involved very gentle control, no more was needed, and a great deal of affection. This gradually restored his self-esteem and gave him the necessary security to make further progress with his growing up. With his therapist he went through the various stages described. These included his anger against his mother for her virtual separation from him during her own time of stress. He was then able to face up to and to share his feelings about the fatal accident. He was then able to reintegrate with this very warm-hearted family.

Donald

From his referral notes Donald should have been one of the most disturbed and potentially dangerous children I have seen. For four months before his admission to my unit he had been in a psychiatric hospital, in an adult male ward occupied by men, many of whom were schizophrenic. I never discovered why Donald at the age of nine should have been thought so dangerous that he was confined in that situation, but clearly it was thought necessary at the time.

The family situation was complex. Donald had an elder brother who was not the son of Donald's father, and there was a younger natural sister to Donald. This was important because the paternal grandparents made a great fuss of Donald and neglected the older brother. This may have been a factor in the mother's rejection of Donald, though the mother's behaviour could not be explained on any rational grounds. Throughout Donald's life, at least until the age of 18, the mother's behaviour to him was extraordinary and inexplicable. She would not have him home for holidays, even Christmas, and there was one Christmas when Donald was the only child in the unit. The staff gave him a wonderful time, but he would have happily done without any of this to be at home. She remained an enigma. She rarely visited the unit, but the social worker visited regularly, although the distance was considerable and involved winter driving over quite hazardous roads. The social workers played a vital role in all cases. Simon's illustrates this very well, but in Simon's case the individual therapy and the skilled handling of the care staff had crucial and quite distinctive roles. The same was true with Iris. In Donald's case the main burden of the therapeutic process lay with the social worker, Elizabeth Brown. In her regular visits to the family she was very supportive to the mother, and in fact supported her through a number of psychotic episodes. During these, the mother heard voices, and on occasion drove too quickly through the local town pursued by the 'Furies'. In spite of the severity of this condition she looked after the rest of the family well. She was a musician, took part in ceilidhs, and at times broadcast on the radio. Donald was extremely unhappy at the long separation from his family. Elizabeth Brown used to have long talks with him following her visits to his home. At times she played him tapes of his mother's music. With his therapist, Donald was never able to express his grief at the separation from his family, nor did he confide in any other members of staff. Although his mother rarely visited or wrote to Donald she tried to dictate how his life was to be run. The children in the unit used to have one afternoon a week to go shopping with their pocket money in the town. At first they would go with a member of staff, but as they became more responsible they could go on their own or with other children. This sometimes had interesting results, as in the case of Jacky (see Chapter 6), and was an essential learning process for many of the children.

The mother would not countenance Donald going out on his own, so I made a home visit. I told the mother that if I had to take full responsibility for Donald I would decide what he could and could not do. If she wanted to take the responsibilities herself she could take Donald home. It was a stormy interview. I thought it better undertaken by me than Elizabeth Brown, but the mother could not face having Donald home and agreed to my proposals.

Elizabeth Brown played a crucial role with Donald as well as his mother. When she returned from a visit with his mother she had a long session with Donald, telling him how things were at home, and playing tapes for him that the mother had recorded. I found this quite painful, the mechanical voice instead of the real thing.

It must be clear by now that Elizabeth Brown played a key role in Donald's therapy. This is not to say that the contribution of the care staff, and other therapists, was not important. They were equally vital in this strange case, and without the care staff and all the other supports Donald could not have survived. But even more than in some of the other cases, this was the sharp end of the therapeutic process.

The time came when Donald was quite capable of moving on to a secondary school. His mother still would not have him at home so with her reluctant approval we found a foster home quite near the unit. After a very short time mother descended on the foster home and effectively destroyed it as a possible residence for Donald. By this time I had moved to Edinburgh. I broke a long-standing rule never to mix work with family and took him into my own home until a place could be found for him in a children's home nearby. Donald was epileptic – the fits easily contained with medication. I continued to be concerned with his care as was Elizabeth Brown. Donald asked me one day if he could stop taking his tablets. I said he could if he maintained certain strict conditions for at least six months, such as not riding a bicycle and not going swimming. Donald did this and had no further trouble.

Elizabeth was interested in horses, and Donald got a job in a stable. His first job was mainly 'mucking out' but then he learned to ride. He made friends locally and was so popular that he was chosen as the 'Lad' for the local Riding of the Marches. This entailed riding at the head of 200 horsemen and women in his red coat, carrying the flag of his town on his stirrup, to hand it back unsullied at the end of the year. Donald's parents came to see the ceremony, but Donald was still not a member of the family.

Donald had a number of jobs in connection with his chosen craft, and eventually landed a very prestigious job indeed. His mother was at last proud of him and he was at long last accepted. Elizabeth Brown remained in touch. She remained an unfailing support not only for Donald but for the whole family as well. Unprofessional? I don't think so. I have thought and thought about this case in terms of all the theoretical models, and I am still thinking about it today.

Agatha

This girl was admitted to Ladyfield when she was ten and a half. She settled in quite well but the staff were always concerned about her. She was not too difficult with the staff but she was most unpleasant with the other children. In Ladyfield there was always an atmosphere of affection towards the children and many of them spent a good deal of time cuddling the staff. Agatha would have none of this. She remained aloof and constantly looked for ways of hurting any children weaker than she was. Her story was a very unhappy one. When she was two and a half she was crawling about the floor and came across a bottle of caustic soda. She swallowed some of this. It burned her throat and she was taken to hospital. The noxious fluid was washed out but the doctors were worried about a constriction of the larynx during the healing process. So at regular and quite short intervals a mercury bougie was pushed down her throat. No instructions were given to the staff about how to approach her or give her any explanation. She was of course very young. The nurses, who hated this procedure, tried to act and appear as pleasant as possible. This meant that sometimes someone approached the child smiling and then did something very nasty and at other times did something nice.

To a child of Agatha's age this meant that adult behaviour made no sense; she was unable to interpret it. We thought that something like this must have happened to make Agatha so impervious to any show of affection or any attempt to get anywhere near her. She was the only child on whom Ladyfield had no beneficial effect. Of the other children, some made dramatic improvements, as has already been described. Others improved but in a less spectacular way. Agatha was the only one with whom we failed completely.

Danny

Danny came to my unit at the age of nine. He had been in a children's home and while there had attempted to take his

18

life by hanging himself from a tree in the garden of the home. The people who knew him there thought that he genuinely wanted to take his life; he had been very unhappy indeed for some time. Danny's troubles had started early in life. His father had been a German prisoner of war who had elected to stay in this country. His wife was an unhappy woman who was frequently taking off from the family.

Paradoxically this would not have been so bad if she had not come back again. This happened several times. After a while the father had found another woman to look after the children. The mother would come back and send the new foster mother packing, and after a short while would disappear again. On one of these occasions Danny, who was four and a half, was found about 20 miles down the road on a child's tricycle, pedalling furiously. He said he was trying to find his mother. Danny's father was very worried about this kind of adventure, so Danny had then been sent to the children's home.

Danny settled surprisingly well in the unit and most weekends he went home to his father. Then his father disappeared and we had no communication with him by letter or phone. After a while Danny became desperate. He said he must try to find his father. I offered to take him by car to the last known address, but he insisted he must go by himself. When I had failed to persuade him otherwise I gave him some money and wished him luck. He returned late in the evening by which time I was very worried. He told me he had gone to the last known address of his father, and a neighbour had told him he had moved and gave him the new address. Danny bought some sweets and some flowers and set off for the new address. His father was there and told him he had been away to another county doing a course connected with his trade. He had come back and had found a new mother for the children. Unfortunately she had a family of her own and there was no room for Danny. This was goodbye for the last time. I was very relieved that Danny came back to me.

Danny settled again surprisingly well in the unit and after a while a foster home was found for him. All went well for a few weeks and then Danny landed back at the unit. Something had gone wrong, and in spite of their promises they never wanted to see him again. Surprisingly he settled again, and then went to a children's home. Danny said he wanted to go into the army so I arranged for him to go to the recruiting office. The major in charge phoned me to say that while he liked the boy they could not take boys of such limited ability. Danny then went to an educational psychologist who helped him greatly to fill some of the gaps in his learning. He was in fact a boy of good intelligence. He then became an apprentice joiner with a good estate. After two and a half years he came to me and said he was going to try again for the army. I tried to dissuade him and said it would be better to finish his apprenticeship first but he persisted and after a short time was accepted by the army and eventually went into the Parachute Regiment. He enjoyed this and his hobby was free-fall diving. He married but this did not last very long.

When he came out of the army he married again and this was more successful. He worked as a joiner for some time but then went back to the army. All this time he kept up a warm friendship with one of the nurses who had helped him while he was in the unit. I think this was a lifeline for him.

It is not easy to define Danny's development in terms of the theoretical models. In the early stages Danny obviously had a strong attachment to his mother. Somehow he was able to make attachments to other people and to thrive on these. So far as cognitive development theory is concerned, he had fallen a long way behind the norms for his age. The army recruiting officer told me that in the aptitude tests they had given him he had scored an all time low. Yet he had been able to catch up and in time reach a high standard, or he would not have been accepted for the Parachute Regiment. This is a remarkable story, and probably shows how a child can survive and achieve considerable success with what seems like very little, but that little has to be of high quality.

Robert

Many children who have a specific difficulty or handicap have a number of other difficulties, which are not directly related to the main problem but can still cause great difficulties for the child. The child I shall describe first had a severe reading difficulty, some call this dyslexia, but dyslexia stands for a number of different conditions, and I prefer to call these conditions 'specific learning difficulties' and then specify the actual difficulties. As will be seen in Robert's case most of his difficulties disappeared when the real problem was recognised and treated.

Robert was referred to me at the age of nine. He was at a private preparatory school. His older brother had been there and had done well and was now at a 'public school'. Robert at nine could neither read nor write but what bothered the school was that he could not even play rugby football. I said that to assess him properly I would have to admit him for a short time to my residential unit.

He was tested in various ways and some remarkable difficulties became apparent. He seemed to have a severe memory defect. If I asked him to get me a cup he would go out of the room muttering 'get the doctor a cup, get the doctor a cup' and if when he got to the door I said 'and please bring me a saucer as well' that threw him completely and he could not do anything. He also seemed to have a degree of spacial disorientation. When he was playing football he often kicked the ball towards his own goal, which made him unpopular

21

with his own side. There were other problems and I finished off with a very complicated diagnostic assessment.

Psychometric testing showed that he had a very severe learning difficulty with regard to reading but in other ways was of superior intelligence. I told Robert that he was one of the brightest boys in the place but he had this particular difficulty and we would find ways to help him. I also told him he could overcome his reading problem but he would have to work hard at it. He stayed with me for two terms by which time we had found out how best to help him. By this time he had increased enormously in confidence and I had crossed out all the items in my complex diagnostic formulation except for 'specific learning difficulty related to reading'. For example, I could now give him a message containing five unrelated items and he would take it accurately to another member of staff and bring back accurately an equally complicated message.

I saw the parents and told them that Robert needed individual treatment by an expert before he was ready to go back to school, but that apart from his reading difficulty he was a bright boy. Their response was 'Thank you very much, doctor, we are so glad to hear that he is really a clever boy', and they sent him straight back to the original preparatory school. Within a term he had regressed to the state he was in when I first saw him. All the secondary symptoms had returned, the memory loss, and so on.

The parents had the good sense to bring him back to me. We arranged for him to be taught at home by a teacher experienced in these problems and he went out to play with the village children. At 14 he went to an agricultural college and then I lost touch with him until one day he arrived at the door of the unit driving a nice little car. He was then successfully running a 600-acre farm. He was going to the big city to be measured for a gun for his 21st birthday and he had dropped in to say 'thank you'.

This problem illustrated very well that emotional problems can cause secondary disabilities, which may present as much difficulty or even more than the actual disability. In this case there was no lack of care or affection, but it took a little while before the family could make the necessary internal adjustments to come to terms with the reality of the situation.

Johnny

These children needed not only affection, they needed control. How this was done is illustrated by the encounter of Johnny with Tam Gibson. Tam was a senior member of the care staff. He was a very big man and if he had to use force could use it very gently. Johnny had a number of problems. He had been expelled from two schools for 'maladjusted children'. He was epileptic but his symptoms were controlled by medication and did not contribute in any way to his disturbance, except that as with a number of children who suffer from epilepsy, or indeed asthma, he had never been subjected to any firm discipline 'in case frustration should bring on one of his fits'. He was 12 when he came to my residential unit, a well-built boy for his age and of good intelligence.

He arrived at the unit in a state of some apprehension. He had an idea that it must be somewhere near the end of the road, and was quite surprised to find that there were no bars on the windows. He spent the first two days getting his bearings. He found that the children talked quite freely to the staff, and even seemed to be cheeky at times. He decided that he could take this place apart rather more easily than any of the other places he had been in. So during one mealtime he started. He kicked one child under the table, upset the one next door to him with his elbow and started throwing food around the room. The decibel level rose alarmingly and chaos was imminent. Tam, who was there, quietly took Johnny under his arm and removed him from the room. On the rare occasion this was necessary: just taking the child outside was usually enough to calm him or her down, and they were able to return and continue their meal without fuss. For Johnny, however, this was a showdown and Tam took him up to one of the bedrooms. Johnny was a little scared at this point. Here was a big man and there was no one near. However, all Tam did was to say, 'I'm sorry, Johnny, you will have to stay with me until you settle down.' Johnny went into a temper tantrum. He raged and swore but all Tam did was to repeat what he had said. He stopped Johnny hurting himself or Tam or from doing any actual damage to the room, although the room looked as if a bomb had hit it. After about 40 minutes they were both a little tired, and they sat down on one of the disordered beds. Johnny said, 'Well you are the first man who has managed to control me.' Tam said to him that perhaps it was a good thing for someone to be able to control him; he was not very old and if no one could control him they would not be able to look after him properly. Johnny thought there might be some sense in this and they talked amiably for a while. Then Johnny said, 'I don't suppose you get many as bad as me.' He had to be the best at being bad. Tam said, 'Well a number of children who come here have to see how far they can go and see what happens.' 'What does happen?' said Johnny. 'Well I don't think anything happens now, I don't think either of us enjoyed that much, I think you had better wash your hands and go down to tea.' This was too much for Johnny. 'You ain't seen nothing yet,' and he went into another temper tantrum. But the steam had gone out of the situation, he was neither a hero nor a martyr. Tam was still in complete control of himself and of the situation. So this lasted only a few minutes. Tam then said, 'Well I think you had better wash your hands again and you might put a comb through your hair.'

After this Johnny had one or two minor tantrums but soon settled to be a reasonable member of the community.

So this was the ultimate method of control. It was rarely used. The relationships between the children and the staff were usually so good that most of the time the children wanted to please the staff.

Punishments were given – simple things like going to bed early. Sometimes if a child was very distressed he or she would be put to bed but always with a member of staff sitting with them. This was a useful therapeutic system.

Occupational Therapists

From the early days of Ladyfield the occupational therapists played a big role in the scheme of things. They undertook the group therapy. This applied to all children and is described in Chapter 2. They also did a good part of the individual therapy. When the second house of the unit was opened I had built a separate building especially for the occupational therapists. This had six rooms and included an office, play rooms, a work room fitted with the tools, and a kitchen, which was very popular with the boys and girls. The occupational therapists became very interested in the therapy. One, Glenys Parkinson, who had done very good pioneer work in Ladyfield, went to Canada where she got into a university, obtained a BA, a Masters degree and then a PhD. Two other occupational therapists who worked in Ladyfield also went off and did degrees and continued practising their therapy at an even more sophisticated level.

It will be seen from the description of some of these children that their effective treatment required a very sophisticated approach by the care staff. The children had great needs for affection and this they got. The staff showed great affection to the children and this was reciprocated. This might seem to be politically unacceptable now, but it was an essential part of the therapeutic process, and many of the metamorphoses described would not have happened without it. It was soon found that if children had feelings of hostility to their parents, as they began to feel secure in the unit, they worked out their hostility on their parent substitutes – the staff. This was hard to take when you had given the child so much affection. When the staff came to realise that this was an important phase in the child's development they coped remarkably well.

There were always male staff on duty and if a girl was being subjected to a degree of anger, which was more than she could really take, a man would come to her rescue. He would not just take over, he would say to the girl, 'Would you mind doing such and such for me?', and thus quietly take over. Care staff had also to learn the role of the 'first best person' and the 'second best person'. Children tended to attach themselves to a particular member of the care staff. When that member was off duty they attached themselves to another. When the original person returned the child would spurn and sometimes be quite nasty to their second choice. This was hurtful but the rejected person needed to understand that this was essential to the child's growth and development. When the child became more secure he or she could accept all members of the staff equally.

It will be seen that this level of sophistication came only with time and with very good communications.

The children's week started on Monday. They went to school each day, and two days a week they went swimming in the hospital pool, which they had to themselves. On one afternoon in the week they went shopping in Dumfries. At first they were accompanied by a member of staff in mufti. Later, when they were thought to be able, they went on their own and spent their pocket money. For all children this was fun and for many a very important experience. All children had individual therapy though only about one third needed intensive therapy like Iris or David. Few children had ever had the experience of a sensible conversation with an adult and this was important for them. All had group therapy once a week. This will be described later.

Equally important was the work with families. This was done mostly by the social worker, though I was closely involved in this and saw all the families at some time. The social workers when they applied for a job in Ladyfield were told that the work involved at least one day in Ladyfield at the weekend when families usually visited. The work also involved a good deal of travelling as some of the families lived at a considerable distance and some were at first reluctant to visit. This is described in more detail in the accounts of the individual cases.

Reviews

One of the most important routines in Ladyfield was the regular review of all the children at the end of each term. This was done under six headings:

Work with the family,
Work with care staff,
Work with the teacher,
Work with the psychologist,
Individual therapy,
Group therapy.

Each person prepared his or her report, came up to a table on which there was a microphone and a tape recorder. So the whole staff shared in the review. Having to record your work like this wonderfully concentrates the mind. At first staff members were apprehensive about this but they learned from other people and very soon were producing reports of a high professional standard. The reports were vivid because the people concerned had actually done the work with the children.

When I was in Edinburgh I used to go to a very good school – Lady Mary. They were familiar with Ladyfield and adopted my system of reviews. I always attended. One day during a review one of the care staff described a child as being pleasant and biddable. A junior member of the care staff burst into tears and said, 'No, he's not like that, he's a little horror and I can't do a thing with him.' After the meeting I went to the girl and said that I thought she had made the most important contribution to the discussion. After this the contribution of the care staff was made by two people, one a senior member and the other one recently joined. This gave a very rounded picture of the child. The first part showed the child's potential with skilled handling while the second gave a vivid picture of what the mother or father was up against.

I met a social worker at some function and he said to me, 'I went to Ladyfield once and it was one of the worst professional experiences of my life.' He said he was looking after a family whose child was in Ladyfield, and he was invited to the review. He went to the meeting and I was a few minutes late. Some of the female staff were knitting. He thought, 'What sort of joint is this?' Then I arrived and the meeting started. He was to see some of those women who had been knitting go up to the table and read out very detailed and professional reports. Then he was asked to make his contribution. He had nothing prepared and stumbled through an ad hoc report. He said he never again went anywhere without doing his homework.

CHAPTER 2

Group Therapy

Group therapy played a very important and quite specific part in treatment of all the children in the unit. In addition to the therapeutic aspect, it made a subtle and significant contribution to the diagnostic procedures. Its main function was that of a controlled therapeutic medium in which the child learns to relate to the adult first in competition with, and later in co-operation with, other children – perhaps the most 'natural' therapeutic situation a residential unit has to offer. It also gave valuable information of prognostic significance, such as when the child was ready to go home, finally, or, as was often done, sending the child home for an extended trial period. These three aspects of group therapy will be discussed in some detail in relation to particular children.

Group therapy differs in several respects from all other situations in which the children found themselves in the unit. The small groups (two to four children) were seen once or twice weekly, at regular times. Twice weekly sessions are always preferable, but often once weekly sessions had to be accepted. The child was never compelled to come to the sessions; children very rarely *refused* to come, though some children went through phases of erratic attendance, clearly related to their relationship with the therapist, or, more rarely, through being anxious about or frightened of the other children. It was never necessary to ensure that a child did something as the care staff had to do – like insisting they go to bed.

It was rarely necessary to frustrate the children in the sense of stopping them doing something, unless what they were doing was dangerous or damaging, and the child almost always accepted such control with relief. The only frustrations they had to accept were occasions such as waiting in turn for the therapist's attention and individual help, or for a tool in use by another child. Such frustrations are clearly related to constantly recurring situations in everyday life. Helping the child to cope with them by patience, understanding and fair dealing are obviously of great importance to a disturbed child and it is the information about the child's behaviour in these situations that is of such value diagnostically and prognostically.

Besides being accepting, the environment in the group session was stimulating. There were interesting things to do, and unlike the school situation there were no fixed standards. Full approval might be given to very slapdash or indifferent work – it may be the first creative effort the child has made since admission. The situation is quite a novel one for the child, and as such is largely uncomplicated by previous attitudes of conformity with or rebellion against school. In the very small groups very warm relationships with the therapist rapidly developed, jealousies and dawning friendships with other children also developed freely in this environment.

There were also obvious differences between the group situation and individual therapy in which there was no competition or interaction with other children. Individual interviews, however valued and however much they may come to mean to the child over a period of time, were in the first instance often frightening. There is some safety in numbers, and during the progress of the group the various members may identify themselves now with the therapist against the children, now with the children against the therapist, or after a time all may work together, friendly, talking freely, and helping each other. It is remarkable that some children find it easier to talk freely in a group than on their own, and in some cases the child's essential attitudes became quite clear from their remarks in the group long before they got round to discussing these things with their therapist, though later on they may have become eager to do this. This is not to decry the value of individual therapy. With any very disturbed children the real heart of the matter often came out in the individual sessions while this was not touched on in the group sessions.

The behaviour of children in a group tends to follow certain recognisable patterns, and superimposed on these can be seen the infinite variations of the child's individual needs and ways of satisfying them in terms of constitutional assets or difficulties, modified by the sum total of past experience. At first each child behaves as an almost isolated individual; their attempts to satisfy their needs bear little relationship with the other children, or to the therapist as a person. These needs are usually simple – something the child wants. The therapist attempts to satisfy these needs, and as the relationship develops the child's behaviour undergoes a marked change. It is now governed mainly by attempts to relate to the therapist in a particular way – the child may want to please the therapist, to annoy the therapist, or to try the therapist out in some direction to see just how far the child can go. The success in handling these problems lies in maintaining an accepting and constructive attitude to each situation as it arises. For example, a child may destroy the work of another child, mainly to 'get back' at the therapist. A lecture on the lines of 'that was not fair' tends to produce further aggressive behaviour on the part of the child, whereas a reaction such as 'I will have to help to put this right' and involving extra attention to the child whose work was damaged makes the point just as clearly and is much better accepted by the children, and the aggressive child soon gets to the stage when they decide that taking it out on the other children is not going to help much. Destructive activity can usually and fairly readily be diverted into something like chiselling or sawing away at a piece of wood, which does not matter. Misuse of tools is countered by quietly removing the tools and locking them up. They can be produced again quite naturally and used safely in a short time, and during the same session. Children feel greater security if they know the adult is in control of the situation. The ultimate sanction is temporary removal of a child from the group by the therapist. If necessary at the unit the male nursing staff were called in. This was a very rare occurrence indeed. A child can usually be readmitted to the group after a few moments. It was not surprising that cooking was one of the most popular occupations in the unit, playing with messy substances and then producing a satisfying result.

When this testing phase has passed – it may be almost non-existent, or it may be fairly severe and prolonged, a warm relationship with the therapist often develops. There are many demands for affection and the child will go out of their way to seek approval and retain it.

Children can go on a long time without relating at all noticeably to other children in the group, but a child can never get away from the fact that they are members of the group, having to share the attention of the therapist and also tools and materials with the other children. At the unit the groups tended to develop an identity very early on. It is quite difficult to introduce a new member to a group and there was often a marked resistance to a change of time – 'We always come at such and such a time.' The development of friendly relations within the group forms a very interesting study, and is of great importance to the children – gradually they begin to show an interest in each other and in each other's work. In some cases a child may work quite happily in an established group at a time when relationships with other children in all other situations are appalling. This emphasises that the dynamics of the group are quite distinct, and the trend of events forms a clearly recognisable thread in the child's experience, a kind of 'counterpoint'. The child's progress can only be followed with any understanding by taking into account all the various aspects of the child's experience.

Michael

An example of the progress of one of the children from a good home is Michael. His problems stemmed from divided authority when he was young, a grandmother who was living with the family always taking his side against the parents. Michael became very skilled at playing people off against each other. He was of superior intelligence, but was not working to his capacity at school. He was truanting. Wandering from home, and stealing. He had no confidence in himself, as his schemes sometimes worked and sometimes brought him trouble. He had no great opinion of adults, and was particularly insecure about female authority. He was continually provoking other children and trying, often unsuccessfully, to set them against each other. He had no means of dealing with the retribution, which periodically descended on him from adults and children, and was a frightened, anxious boy.

When he first joined a group, with three other boys, he was pleased to come, and was very quiet and passive at first, conforming readily to demands of other members of the group. At this stage the therapist made no demands on him, offering him things to do, and helping when he needed help, with some protection from the others.

His behaviour was quite good, and he appeared to be attempting to conform to the standard he had anticipated would be expected of him. However, his concentration was poor, and he seemed to have difficulty in mastering techniques, which were obviously well within his capacity, and which, in fact he later acquired readily. He appeared to want to be mischievous, but to be very uncertain of the reaction of the therapist.

At this point the conduct of the therapy could follow a number of different lines. The option could be to run a comparatively well organised class for craft work, at which the main therapeutic aim is to develop habits of concentration and persistence in an environment that is friendly, not too demanding, but at the same time makes considerable demands on a child. Such an approach to class work is probably the most appropriate one if occupational therapy is undertaken in, for example, an orthopaedic hospital. The other main approach to the problem is to allow the group to develop along the lines dictated by its own internal dynamics, to allow each child to work out his or her own problems in relation to the therapist and the other children. This does not involve a 'totally permissive atmosphere' – such a state, if it existed, would be a chaotic one, frightening to both therapist and child. There can be no security without some definition. In this case the limits set do not permit damage to persons or tools, and define the time and place of the session, and the constitution of the group. Within these limits a wide scope of activity is possible, ranging from craft work of a fair standard to periodic quite messy and unorganised play with clay and other materials with only an occasional reference to constructive activity.

Michael's therapy, as with most children in the unit, followed the second of the two lines described above. The next phase was one of greater capacity for work when he did work, but mixed with a great deal of sly and surreptitious behaviour, and occasionally destructive activity. On one occasion he had to be thrown out, but always returned in good spirits.

As the aggressive phase grew to a close, Michael became demonstratively affectionate, and such 'trying out' of the therapist was much more open, less underhand, and although he was cheeky and at times defiant, he was friendly and cheerful. On one or two occasions he even helped to restrain the others when they were going too far with some rather hectic play.

It is noticeable that during the phases just described Michael was going through similar phases with the nursing staff, only these were more violent. He was very frightened of the other children, and was continually tale-telling to members of the staff with subsequent retribution from the other children. He continually tried to set both children and adults against each other. His relationship in the group with the children as with the therapist, although still precarious, was better than in any other field of activity at that time, and there is no doubt that the adjustments he made and what he learned in this small group helped very substantially towards the eventual satisfactory adjustment in all fields. The striking changes that took place were much greater confidence in dealing with other children and steadily increasing affection to the therapist, and with it an increasing desire to conform to her wishes. He still had periods of destructive behaviour, but had increasing control over these wild episodes; trying out various dodges, at first maliciously, later humorously; his persistence and concentration improved but remained variable.

Mary

Another example of a child who showed very marked differences between her behaviour in the group and that outside is Mary. This child, after very sordid experiences in a very disrupted and sordid home background, was sent to a children's home run by nuns. She was always difficult, and by the time she was nine or ten they could no longer cope with her in the home or in the school.

When she came to the unit she was violent, abusive and

impulsive, always hitting the headlines with outbursts of outrageous behaviour. In striking contrast was her behaviour in a small group, with sympathetic handling by the therapist. Throughout this time she was sweet, affectionate, biddable, and kind and generous to the other children. The contrast between her behaviour there and the hectic course through which she eventually fought her way towards a reasonable adjustment in the larger world could not have been more dramatic, and there was no doubt that the comparative peace she found in the small group was of great importance in developing her capacity for giving and receiving affection and approval, so vital in the rehabilitation of an institutional child.

To sum up, the basis for group therapy may be defined as:

1) Liking for children, and a desire to help them – this must be the basis of a therapeutic relationship.
2) Bringing certain skills and certain materials.
3) Understanding of children's problems. A good deal of detail about the child's problems is essential as a guide to the handling of the child – for example, a child's behaviour may be rude, cheeky or difficult in various ways. It is difficult to sympathise without considerable understanding of the stresses to which the child has been subjected. This is particularly important when the disturbance includes cruelty to other children, which is particularly hard for adults to tolerate. The child who is being bullied must be protected and this offers no problem to the therapist, sympathy being the natural response to the situation; support and reassurance to the bully is much harder to do though sometimes even more necessary. The 'correction' of the bully can form an all-too-easy outlet for the aggression of the therapist.

There are also certain key therapeutic goals:

1) Establishing a warm relationship with the child on which future handling will be based.
2) Through that relationship with the child, helping him or her to accept a share of adult attention, to accept frustration, and later to get on with other children, or at least recognise the importance of other children's aims.
3) Giving children a sense of achievement in the work completed. Unstinted approval may be given to poor work, which may be the first constructive activity the child has shown.
4) Establishment of a sense of responsibility – for example, in the use of tools. There are few other situations in treatment in which this element of trusting the child can be given and the response so readily observed.
5) Establishment of the child's self-confidence in a group situation. The child can feel relatively free, gaining support from the therapist and from the other children. This situation is not so threatening for a very anxious child as is an individual session.
6) Close links with others working with the child, and a knowledge of the stages reached by the child in other situations, is essential.

It is sometimes necessary to remove a child from the group if he or she is disrupting it beyond a point where it can be tolerated. The frequency of use of this ultimate sanction will vary with the experience and resilience of the therapist. In practice it is rarely used. If a child is very anxious they will need a lot of reassurance when they return. If the child is just trying it out then that child can be cheerfully thrown out and as cheerfully readmitted. No adult should ever feel they are shut up with a group of disturbed children with no outlet. Close co-operation with other staff members is necessary for many reasons, one being the child's tendency to play off adults against each other and to try to obtain from one what they have been refused by another.

It is also necessary for the therapist to be aware of the family situation. In the relaxed atmosphere of the group a child may suddenly make comments on an aspect of family affairs that has not previously been discussed with anyone. These comments may be cryptic and allusive, provoked by a remark by another child, and without inside information vital clues may be missed.

Within this framework many opportunities present themselves. Apart from the purely therapeutic aims, diagnostic procedures using these techniques can be of great value – the emotional disturbances and with these combined with some physical disability, as with David (see Chapter 5). These techniques are also very relevant in the investigation and treatment of psychotic and autistic children but this is outside the scope of this account of group therapy.

An Earlier Episode

One of my earliest experiences of group therapy was when I was at the Maudsley Hospital. I was at that time ward registrar and the childcare expert and psychotherapist Mrs Barbara Dockar-Drysdale visited on a Wednesday afternoon. Dr Kenneth Cameron, my boss, instructed me to keep Mrs Dockar-Drysdale amused. I talked with her about what she would like to do. We decided that puppet plays would keep the children and ourselves amused. There was a puppet theatre and the plan of campaign was to focus on the problems of one child. The children of the residential unit all assembled in one room. Mrs Dockar-Drysdale manipulated the puppets aided by one of the male nurses, who, like everyone else, soon fell under her spell. The staff were in the room sitting with the children, often with one or more children on their knee. There was always one staff member very close to the child whose story was being played out. This staff member relayed this child's comment to the puppeteers, so the child saw his or her story being played out.

A typical play would go like this: When the curtain went up a family of father, mother, a boy and a girl would be on the stage. There would be a lot of argument and eventually the father would say, 'I am fed up with this, I am going to the pub.' The mother would retire to the kitchen in tears and the boy and girl would be left alone on the stage. They would talk about things and the boy would say, 'I'm fed up with this, I am going to run away.' The girl would try to dissuade him but in the end off he would go. The next scene would show him all by himself in the street. He would say to the audience, 'I'm hungry, what shall I do?' Various suggestions would come from the audience like 'Pinch the money off the paper stall.' He goes off and a policeman appears. He asks the children, 'Have you seen a little boy on the street?' Some children say 'Yes,' some try to help the boy, some try to get him into trouble. Others say 'No.' When the policeman asks them which way the boy went, some say one way, some the other, for equally mixed motives. The boy has some more adventures and eventually lands up at home and a happy ending is contrived.

Mrs Dockar-Drysdale had wit, humour and a vivid imagination and the whole episode was great fun. Audience participation was a hundred per cent. Members of the staff, as I have said, were sitting with the children and they reported the responses of the different children to the various episodes and this was fed back to the children's therapists.

Sometimes children not in the residential unit were invited to attend. One boy, older and much more sophisticated than the majority of the children came at my instigation. I explained to him what was going on and that children tended to distort the stories in relation to their own problems. I told the boy I wanted his account as a kind of benchmark against which the other versions could be measured. He readily agreed. When he came to write out his story it turned out to be one of the most distorted stories I had seen, the distortions clearly related to his own problems. I always thought this was a valuable therapeutic tool.

CHAPTER 3

Work with Families

Work with families is an essential part of any treatment strategy for a child. This includes, or should do, working with the parent substitutes of a child in care. This is described in Chapter 6.

Case work has been described as the art in which knowledge of the science of human development together with skill in the understanding of the complexities of human relationships are used to mobilise the capacities of the individual, and the resources of the community to bring about a better adjustment between the client and his or her environment. This means the mobilisation of the individual and of appropriate community resources. The community resources may be stretched and their mobilisation difficult.

One of the difficulties is that the family may not see themselves as needing help, or if they do see it, they are very reluctant to admit it. All too often the child has been identified as the source of all the trouble. If their own responsibility has been suggested to them they may be resentful, and the anger they feel toward the child enhanced.

The first task will be to get the trust of the family. This may take some time. Trust is a matter of experience and there is no short cut. It is important for parents to feel that you are on their side. The whole of the early stages of the relationship with parents is better focused on them, what it has felt like to them, the worries they have had, and any resentment they may have against education authorities or anyone else they may have encountered before they came to you. You may well in the early stages be invested with some of this resentment. Anything they may contribute about the child will be of great importance but more progress will be made if the focus initially is on the parents and how they see things.

If the child does well in your care the parents will be relieved and pleased, but then it may dawn on them that if someone else is doing well with their child perhaps they did not do too well themselves. I used to say on these occasions that we have not produced the good things they see in the child, we have merely provided an environment, which the child needed at that time in order to produce the good things he or she had, which came from the family. This may lead to a discussion as to how the parents can move towards meeting the child's needs rather better. Here it is important to help the parents to mobilise their own resources, hopefully on their own initiative. They need to be helped to reach their own conclusions and to try out ways that they see to be relevant. In trying to help people along this road it is important to let people go at their own pace, which may seem to the case worker too slow. You have to be as far as possible non-judgemental with real tolerance. Adults have limited capacity for change, but often quite a small movement will give the child room to grow and to develop ways of behaving that are less destructive to that child and family. Tolerance does not mean altering one's own values, but it does mean acceptance of things as they are, with the expectation that in time they will be different.

I will begin by describing the work with families in my residential unit. Parents who can no longer manage their children, or who are worried about some inexplicable phase in their development are often more angry with the child, though they also have a feeling of guilt. In any case the child is the 'identified patient'.

42

When parents came to me I did not at once undertake to cure their child for them. I tried to reach a consensus with them that here is a problem and we are going to set out together to try to find a solution to it. I saw all parents at some stage or other, and in some cases I undertook the major part of the therapy with them, but most of the work was done by the social workers. They were very skilled and they had to travel very considerable distances. I used to negotiate with them in their interview for the job, that they would normally expect to work on one day in the weekend and have another day off during the week. This worked remarkably well even in the case of married men with families.

These were the people most concerned with families, but all members of staff and especially care staff were 'workers with families'. It was of the utmost importance that any member of a family who visited the unit should feel welcome as though they were part of the show and a very important part at that.

Freddy

The work in my unit involved in most cases long-term and often intensive work with families. In rare cases little or no real work with families was possible, and in a few of these there was a good outcome. One of these was Freddy. He was said to have been the child of an American soldier, not uncommon during the war years. The parents did not marry. The mother then married and had another family. When I first saw Freddy he was eight. He had apparently developed normally during the first few years but during the last two to three years he had regressed to a totally baby level. He would not speak, he wet and soiled himself, and he had taken to eating by pushing food into his mouth. During his stay in the unit Freddy steadily improved. His speech came back and he would eat normally. His wetting and soiling ceased, and in all respects he was behaving like a normal boy of his age. Not surprisingly he was some way behind with his school work but he was quite keen to pick up, and with a lot of help in the small classes we had, there was every reason to think that he would eventually catch up to the low average level forecast by psychometric testing. In the meantime the family had not been neglected. Several home visits had been made, but all attempts to persuade the mother to visit the unit had failed. Then one day she did come and she was to take Freddy home for a long weekend. I saw her on this occasion and told her of Freddy's progress, but she obviously did not believe any of this. I watched them go up the drive to the unit, each walking on opposite sides of the drive, looking at each other suspiciously as they went along. I then saw the mother when she brought Freddy back. I was a little apprehensive about this but she said immediately, 'Isn't Freddy great now, how soon can we have him home?'

Improvement under any treatment can produce dramatic changes in the child and this may induce welcome changes in the family and in their attitude to the child, but this cannot be expected, and more often the child's behaviour in the unit could be good but when he or she went home the old patterns of behaviour and relationships in the family reasserted themselves and it is to counteract this that work with the family is necessary. In terms of systems theory there needs to be a reorientation within the family and this, in most cases, needs work of varying intensity with the family. Expecting the child to do all the work, as with Freddy, is not often a viable option.

As I have said, in most cases work with families was intensive for most children in the unit. This was necessary because in the majority of cases the trouble started and was continued by things that were happening in the family. With the autistic children there was no evidence that family problems

44

had anything to do with the onset or development of the autistic condition. But having an autistic child is a situation of great stress for all members of the family and they needed all the help that could be given them.

Examples of the work with families are given in the stories of Simon, Donald and Robert, featured in Chapter 1. In Simon's case there was a considerable distance from the home to the unit, but the work with the family was very intense and in every way similar to what would have been done with a family nearer at hand. The way the family became involved is described and how their trust was gradually secured. Particularly important was the involvement of the father, initially quite hostile to any involvement and the fact that the mother, who at first was very lacking in confidence, gradually asserted herself and came to take an equal part in the discussions, her views being accepted as of equal weight with those of the father, which had never previously been the case in their marriage.

In the case of Donald, the work with the family was of equal intensity, though done mostly at a distance, and there was, after a long time, an equally happy outcome. In this case the mother was supported through a number of psychotic episodes by the very skilled work of the social worker, and she held things together after Donald had left the unit.

Also described in Chapter 1 are the families of Iris and Danny. The outcome in these cases was the break up of the family, but the support and affection given to the children was enough to give them the security they needed in order to lead full lives and to engage in long-term and satisfactory relationships with others.

Dennis

One of the most striking cases I have seen that illustrates the importance of families was a boy called Dennis. He was one of six children. Both parents had been to prison for neglect of the children. When they came out efforts were made to reunite the family. The mother was sent with the two youngest children to a special unit designed to help mothers who had previously failed with their families. Conditions in the family did not improve and the parents separated. The children were taken into care. The places available were limited and the children were each placed in a different children's home, widely separated.

Dennis was thought to be the most difficult, and when it seemed that no home could contain him he came to my unit. He was then eleven, and showed himself to be aggressive, bullying younger children, and he was also aggressive and thoroughly unpleasant with the staff. He was very difficult to give affection to. Attempts were made to link up with the parents. With the mother this was particularly difficult: she was living with her parents and doing odd jobs. The father was unemployed and lived in a single bare room. When the social worker visited, he showed no interest in the family, and on one occasion when she was talking with him he got up without a word, picked up his mackintosh and walked out, leaving her in that bare room. She persisted and eventually she persuaded him to visit the unit. He arrived on the doorstep and by chance Dennis was at the other end of the hallway. To everyone's surprise they rushed into each other's arms.

The change in Dennis as a result of this visit was dramatic. He became a much nicer boy, got on well with the other children and was pleasant and biddable with the staff. It was arranged that he would go to one parent or the other, usually the father, each alternate weekend.

It was then possible for Dennis to go on to a children's home and I laid great emphasis on the importance of his contact with the family. The social work department thought otherwise. They looked at the family's awful record and decreed that there should be no contact with them. Very soon

Dennis set fire to the school he attended, doing several thousand pounds worth of damage. By this time I had moved to Edinburgh, and Dennis was outside the catchment area of my hospital. However, I admitted him to the residential unit and sent him to the family on the first weekend. He travelled there and back on his own. He soon settled down and was able to go to a more understanding children's home where they kept up the regular contact with the family. I followed him up for some time and he never looked back.

Since the writing of John Bowlby – eminent British psychiatrist and psychoanalyst – the importance of the family has been recognised, but this has led in some cases to leaving children in situations where they were at risk, and some children have lost their lives as a result of this, as well as suffering extreme cruelty. In Dennis's case there was no way the parents could care for him, but the contact with them was essential to his well-being. I have described other children where contact with the parents has broken down completely, and in these cases it takes a great deal to fill this gap, although it can be done given loving and entirely dependable parent substitutes. Iris (Chapter 1) and Cynthia (Chapter 9) are good examples of this.

Family Therapy

When I hear of family therapy I always ask who is doing it. I have seen some of the pioneers of this important tool and their methods were very different. First I worked with John Bell. He was a genuine pioneer, in fact he could be said to have initiated family therapy as such. He read a paper by John Bowlby in which he said that in dealing with families when he became stuck he sometimes saw the whole family together for one or two sessions. John Bell thought he meant he was seeing all the family all the time. So he tried it.

When he told Bowlby about this Bowlby said he had never thought of trying this. John Bell was a very quiet man who could hold a group together, giving each member a feeling that they all mattered and that their views and their feelings would all be taken into account. John Bell did not ask for families who presented 'good therapeutic prospects'. In fact he asked for some of the most difficult and deprived families, as did Minuchin in some of his work. The results of Bell's work were impressive.

I then saw American author and psychotherapist Virginia Satir in action. She always made me think of the Great Earth Mother. She was very skilled at making people feel not just at home, but as though they lived in a great caring world where people were there to help other people. She too produced noted results and because she was such a charismatic character attracted more attention than John Bell. Then there was Salvadar Minuchin, the Argentine family therapist. He was a big man and a big personality. He gave a role-playing demonstration at a hospital at which I worked. One of the social workers was to be the mother. One of the consultants, a woman, was rather miscast as the adolescent boy, and one of the doctors was the father. Minuchin arranged the family in a row on chairs. He sat down next to 'mother' and with his back to the rest of the family. 'Mother' had been told her role was to dominate all conversations and she played up well. Then Minuchin asked her what the father thought about it. 'But he never says,' said the mother. 'What about the boy?' 'He never says either.' Minuchin then moved his chair out a little and turned to the boy, puffing at a cigarette so that a smoke screen was produced between him and the mother. He then moved to the other side of the boy and started talking to the father. Mother and boy began to talk together. This was a very vivid and humorous demonstration but I thought you would need to be a Minuchin or something like it to carry it off.

There are many forms of family therapy and it is a most useful tool, but it does need skilled training for the practitioners. I have been involved in various forms of family therapy. In one case it was a family of six children living unhappily in a high rise building. The therapy was done jointly with a social worker. We visited the flat weekly in the evening. There was no way we could get the whole family to the clinic. We made a point of sitting at right angles to each other. In our discussions afterwards there were three different types of information. One where we both saw or heard the same incident and each put the same interpretation on it. Another when we both experienced the incident but put different interpretations on it, and a third piece of data when only one of us noticed it. Although we were both very experienced we found it helpful to be supervised by a third person.

Family therapy was an important ingredient in the therapy of many families I have tried to help.

Parenting

No discussion of work with families would be complete without reference to the fairly recent studies on parenting. One of the more interesting studies was published in 1994 by Puckering, Rogers, Mills, Cox and Mattsson-Graff. This was based on an intervention offered to mothers based on a multidimensional model of parenting developed during a study of Newpin, a volunteer-befriending project aimed at helping mothers in a deprived inner-city area. Observational measures of parenting were derived by the research group from the current literature and previous research. These were validated experimentally, showing coherent interrelationships and a correspondence with child behaviour problems. The dimensions were autonomy, anticipation, warmth and stimulation, co-operation, emotional containment and control. The work was done at the Alloa Family Centre, managed by John Rogers.

The intervention programme involved the mothers volunteering to join the group. It also involved video recordings of the interaction of the mothers and their children in their own homes. One of the striking findings was that mothers at the end of the project felt that they had gained most from the contributions of the other mothers rather than from the professionals involved. The whole tenor of the project was to try to help mothers to find resources in themselves, and it involved exploration of their relationships with their children rather than anyone telling them what to do.

I was interested in this project for several reasons. I was interested in the approach to the mothers as described above, and I was interested in the use of videos. One of the great difficulties in attempting to describe human behaviour is that verbal descriptions are inadequate, as people use words like 'warmth' in so many different ways. A video at least provides material that can be discussed and evaluated.

This brief account cannot do justice to this careful piece of work, but it is quoted to illustrate the importance of parenting in current thinking and some of the work which is going on. Attachment theory lays great emphasis on parenting, but it has so far had too little impact on current teaching.

CHAPTER 4

Epilepsy

Epilepsy is a manifestation of dysfunction of the central nervous system, and is manifested by the patient having fits. These may take various forms. One of the most common is known as 'grand mal'. This involves the patient having a fit which consists of convulsions of a large part of the musculature. There is in most cases a characteristic electroencephalogram. Another common form is 'petit mal' in which there are no convulsions. The patient stops what he or she is doing, has a moment of blankness, and then carries on, not always aware of the area of blankness. This also has a characteristic EEG with 'spike and wave' patterns. There are many other forms of epilepsy. It must be emphasised that the diagnosis of epilepsy is a clinical one. While many have this characteristic EEG pattern, this is not invariable, and there are some people who have an EEG pattern suggestive of epilepsy but who never have fits.

I will describe some cases.

John

John was referred to me at the age of ten. The letter from the family doctor said: 'This boy has intractable epilepsy. The paediatricians have failed to control his fits and a place has been arranged for him in an epileptic colony. He is such a difficult boy at home that I thought you might take him in to your unit until the place in the epileptic colony becomes available.' I was not very flattered by this referral but I took the boy in. The epilepsy was of an interesting kind. His fits involved stopping what he was doing making a few apparently random movements of his head and body. If he was standing up he did not fall down. The most disturbing series of events followed. He had a period lasting up to two minutes of post-ictal automatism. One occasion when he was at home he had walked out into the traffic on the road and on another occasion he had walked into the river, which luckily was shallow. It was these episodes that had alarmed the family. John was one of a family of six children. It was an efficient family and none of the other children had either epilepsy or any kind of behaviour disorder.

When John came in to the unit he showed himself to be a very awkward, self-willed boy, obviously used to having his own way in everything. After some early struggles with the staff he settled down and obviously felt more secure in an orderly, predictable environment where he had reasonable freedom and where his own wishes, though not always immediately implemented, were respected. I took him off his drugs and only attempted to control his fits when he was himself settled into a sensible regime. After this, it was not difficult to find the medication that suited him and that controlled his fits. As long as he was in the unit he was well controlled both in his behaviour and his fits. When he went home the fits recurred. It took several weeks before the parents could bring themselves to treat him like the other children, expecting the same compliance as the other children and the same freedom. Over the years they had regarded him as someone special who needed a special sort of treatment quite different from other 'normal' children. This tends to lead to a situation in which the parents' tolerance is stretched at an unpredictable time to the limit. When the limit is reached almost inevitably they come down hard on the child. The child therefore lives in an unpredictable world in which he or she is constantly testing to find where the limits are. I am sure from observation of a number of cases that this anxiety and uncertainty makes it more likely that the fits recur. It was only when at last they were persuaded to treat John as normal that he did behave normally: This is a common pattern with epileptic children. Eventually, when the parents and the boy had learned this lesson, the boy was able to go home.

I followed him up in out-patients for some time and then lost touch with him. Then I remembered him and wrote a letter to his head teacher asking about him. Usually I am more discreet about these things. I had a letter back, which said, 'I see from the letter heading that this boy has been under your care. I can't think why. He is doing well in school and plays for the school football team. He obviously had some difficulties when he was in primary school because when he came to this school he was functioning well below his true level. He has now nearly caught up. I hope this is what you wanted to know.' It was very much what I wanted to know about a boy who had been written off.

The pattern this boy showed I saw in several children referred to me. I was successful in treating these children largely because I treated them myself, and became aware quite early on of the very large psychological element that comes with these children. The same problem is often seen in children with asthma. The parents think the child has to be coddled and cannot cope with the same discipline as 'normal' children. The attachment pattern is distorted. Cognitive development is often impeded. With regard to systems theory it is essential for parents to reorganise their thinking with regard to the child, and they often need to support each other in this.

Malcolm

Malcolm came to me at the age of eleven. He was epileptic and had been asked to leave two preparatory schools. He was then regarded as ineducable, as in addition to his fits and quite severe behaviour disorders resulting from the many frustrations he had suffered, he had a severe learning difficulty, specifically related to reading and writing. He was admitted to the in-patient unit and investigations were carried out. These revealed a very severe learning difficulty, but a very high potential. This was before the days when computers were readily available, and some of the earlier teaching was done using felt letters on a felt pad. Malcolm made good progress, and after a year was able to go to a good preparatory school. From there he went to a good public school. Surprisingly, in spite of his learning disability, especially in reading and writing, he had a great aptitude for classical language. When it came to his A-levels I wrote a long report specifying precisely his difficulty. He was given an extra hour for each paper and did well.

He was admitted to a good university where the pastoral care was good. When it came to his degree exams, he was given only an extra half hour for each paper. He obtained third class honours, but he had completed only half of each paper. However, so good were the halves he had done that he was asked to stay on and do a PhD. This was pretty good for a boy who had once been written off educationally.

Derek

Derek was another such case, He showed problems with the family similar to those of John. The family was a very stable and caring one. The father did a skilled and responsible job. Derek was a lively energetic toddler, and one day when he was four he got out on the road and was hit by a car. The parents felt responsible for this and from that time onwards were overprotective towards Derek. When Derek developed epilepsy they were even more upset. Derek became very difficult to handle and was admitted to my unit. His epilepsy was more straightforward than that of John and in the unit was easily controlled, but at home the fits persisted. With some parents there would have been a suspicion that the medication was not being given regularly, but not with these careful and caring people. In terms of systems theory they had become so obsessed with their guilt and the resulting overprotection that it was several weeks before they could bring themselves to exercise the firm but kindly discipline the child needed. When they achieved this the fits stopped at home as well as in the unit.

Albert

Another boy who was in danger of overprotection was Albert. I saw him as an out-patient. He had major fits, which responded well to treatment. He said to me one day, 'My mother says I must not do sport now.' I asked if he was keen on sport and he said he was. I told him that as long as he took his medication regularly he could carry on with his sport. He said that the sport he liked best was athletics. I saw him about three months later. He said things were going well. I remembered to ask him if he had gone on with his sport. He was quite modest but when I pressed him he said that at the recent meeting he had broken four county records. I did not hear about him for some years but one evening at about 10 p.m. his mother phoned. She said I must mostly get bad news late at night, but she had phoned me to tell me that the boy had just obtained his degree.

There are some other points I would like to make. There is a danger that when a child attends an out-patient department he or she may be seen by a variety of doctors. One boy of 15 I saw in a residential school had major fits and was put on medication. He was always unwilling to take this. Then he came back from a visit to the hospital saying that the doctor had said he did not have epilepsy. I wrote to the consultant asking for a report. To my surprise they sent me the file of their notes. These showed that he had been seen originally by the consultant but on subsequent visits by a series of junior doctors, one of whom had said he did not have epilepsy. It was quite difficult to persuade the boy to continue with his medication.

I was always insistent on recording the exact number of fits and the time at which they occurred. With difficult cases I allocated a staff member to be with the child for 24 hours and to record each fit and the time. When I was in New Zealand a professor said that my methods were out of date. They used time samples. Although this method was statistically sound they used to argue about how many fits a child had had, which never happened in my unit. Only if you have all the data can you prescribe accurately the medication and the timing of it.

Margaret

I had only one adult patient at this time. Her name was Margaret. She and her husband came to me in some distress. The man was considerably older than his wife and he attended a clinic, which had its own quite strict rules. It was totally against all forms of traditional medicine and particularly against any form of conventional drugs. His wife was epileptic. The husband took her to his clinic. They told the family that she should think of herself as a second-class citizen. She should give up her work and not have a family. The newly married couple were not happy about this and came to me as a person they could trust. I persuaded them to try an anticonvulsant medicine. They said that any drug would have a devastating effect on her. I gave her a very small dose of the most innocuous of the anticonvulsants and she was prostrated, sick, and feeling awful for three days. They said to me that they had predicted this. I said we had not tried all the options and I was going to play a trick on them. I would give her a powder and at first it would have no drug in it and then one day I would add the drug. A co-operative pharmacist made up a number of powders and for ten days there was no drug. Then I scraped a minute quantity of the drug into the powder. I gradually increased this until in about a month she was having a full dose. After another month I told them how it had gone. I said I had every confidence that she was now free from the risk of fits and could and should lead a normal life. She continued her job and had four healthy children. The clever part of this was not the little trick I played on them with the drug but the fact that I was able to keep their faith in their clinic intact. The lifestyle the clinic prescribed was a healthy one and belief in the clinic was very much part of their faith.

This happy story illustrated very well another aspect of the psychological problems associated with epilepsy.

CHAPTER 5

Organic Disorders of the Central Nervous System

It has always been my view that many conditions seen in childhood have as their origin an element of dysfunction of the central nervous system (CNS). These include infantile autism, schizophrenia, specific learning difficulties (including dyslexia, a term I am reluctant to use to specify the difficulty) and epilepsy, which has already been dealt with.

In many cases disabilities originating in the central nervous system (CNS) are exacerbated by further disabilities of psychological origin. I have called these the Grey Areas, and they have been described in the case of Robert (Chapter 1), and in other children. In other cases where there is more severe dysfunction of the CNS the child may be helped to overcome these real difficulties by intensive treatment. Such a case is that of David, described below. Some of his treatment is given in detail, because it illustrates very well how cut off a child can become when he has this kind of organically based disability, and how long it can take to connect that child up again, and the effort required.

Rather similar problems can be found when the treatment of autistic children is undertaken. In virtually all these cases there is a psychological element, in that the child, as it attempts to relate to other children, or to adults, finds real difficulty, and this can discourage the child from making further efforts, and may drive him or her further into his or herself. In many cases, effective treatment can help a child to come much nearer to reaching his or her potential. This treatment is, however, time consuming and requires skill and great patience from the staff.

Doris

Some diseases of organic origin can present as psychological disorders. One very striking example was Doris, a girl of nine who was in a hospital about 50 miles from my own base. The paediatrician thought Doris was psychotic while the parents thought she had been abused and were shocked by this. When I saw the child she was in bed with her distraught parents at the bedside. She babbled continuously, some sentences reasonably complete and some not. She moved about constantly and frequently rubbed her vulva, which was why the parents were thinking about abuse.

I told the paediatrician that I was sure the condition was not psychotic but had an organic basis. They said that whatever the condition was they could not cope with it in their ward and would I take the child in to my own unit. Reluctantly I agreed, reluctantly because it is not easy to nurse a very sick child in a unit for very disturbed children.

In my unit the child's condition steadily deteriorated, and she lost one function after another until the only one left was her breathing. She could not swallow, and had to be fed with a nasal tube. Fortunately my staff were skilled. By this time the diagnosis was clear, a nasty form of meningo-encephalitis, probably of viral origin. After a few days to my surprise she began to improve, regaining her bodily functions, but as yet with no speech. Then, one day a female nurse was singing a nursery rhyme to her while the girl sat on the nurse's knee. To the nurse's surprise the child finished the line of the nursery rhyme. The improvement continued slowly, until the child was functioning normally. She went home to her very happy parents and I kept in touch. A few years later I had a letter from her father telling me that the girl had passed five O-levels. The child might have recovered under any circumstances but I thought the chances of recovery were enhanced by the staff's amazing tolerance of all aspects of a child's behaviour and their outstanding skills in nursing. Tolerance in this case was not permissiveness. It was an acceptance of the child as she is but with a firm conviction that in the course of treatment the child will be very different.

David

David first came to the unit when he was five. He was presenting a very difficult problem at home. He was retarded in his development, his speech was poor, nasal, high-pitched, monotonous and loud. The content was like that of a much younger child. He was very demanding of attention and reacted with severe temper tantrums to mild frustration. He did not get on at all well with other children and was much teased by them.

He had been a premature baby weighing three and a half pounds at birth. He was in an incubator for the first four weeks of his life and was a further four weeks in hospital before going home. His milestones were passed late. He sat at 11 to 12 months and walked at 22 months, said phrases at three but did not say sentences until four and a half.

At the time of referral his mother and father were separated. The mother was working and needed to pass some very difficult exams in order to continue with her profession. Later there was a messy divorce and David was in the unit longer than was usual. This was partly because of the family situation, but as time went on it became clear that David had a very unusual condition of cerebral dysfunction and it was unlikely that at that time he would have had the intense individual attention needed for his rehabilitation elsewhere. During David's stay in the unit his mother worked full time. The siblings could be looked after by carers but David presented too many problems and had a need to come to terms with a world he had great difficulty in understanding.

When David was first admitted to the unit he was tested for deafness at the local hospital, and was found to be normal. I was never sure about this and after a little time had him tested again, with the same result. After another year he was tested again and this time a quite severe deafness affecting mainly the higher frequencies was found. I do not think these conflicting results were the result of ineptitude on the part of the hospital. David was very difficult to communicate with at this time. On the occasion of the final testing it was found that David was very good at lip reading.

Another investigation, which was routine in the unit, was an electroencephalogram. This showed a marked abnormality. This consisted of 'much spiking activity in both temporal areas. This activity consisted of sharp waves rather than spikes.' The electroencephalographer commented that David would be 'unlikely to be able to use the temporal neurones and there should be a marked disorder of speech.' The disorder was considered to be epileptic in character and he was treated with anticonvulsant therapy. The clinical impression was that his alertness and hearing were considerably improved. The EEG finding did suggest quite severe brain dysfunction and this was shown in his therapy sessions. In these he showed not only difficulty in speech but also in understanding, so that compared with other children of his age and even with children who had a greater degree of hearing loss than he had, a great deal of the ordinary world was a closed book to him.

A report from Dr T.S.S. Ingram of the Royal Hospital for Sick Children in Edinburgh stated that 'This boy shows minimal signs of chronic brain abnormality in that his co-ordination is poor and there are mild pyramidal signs on the left side. These are associated with high tone hearing loss and retarded speech development.'

61

Psychometric testing showed an almost average score on performance items, but he began to fail the verbal items at around a four-year-old level. It was striking that in the *Goodenough-Harris Drawing Test* he scored at an age of six when his chronological age was five years, five months. The psychologist summarised the test as follows:

> Although on formal testing David appears to be functioning at an educationally sub-normal level higher results on performance tests suggest his ability is higher. Most of his failures on verbal items may be explained by his receptive difficulties – i.e. difficulty in grasping the meaning of information fed to him, and this led to an under-estimation on the IQ tests. His attainments are very low for his age, which, again, is probably due to his receptive difficulties plus his distractibility.
>
> David's bright personality plus his occasional spurts of high motivation, however, will probably be a great asset to him. The first in sorting out any social problems, and the second in pushing up his attainments with individual patient coaching.

For this child the beginning part of the individual therapy has been given in some detail. This illustrates David's problems and also gives an idea of the scope of the individual therapy in the unit. In this case it was undertaken by one of the occupational therapists.

Individual Therapy

David was seen for three-quarters of an hour sessions, three times a week: This account of his therapy is in three monthly intervals, taken from end of term reports. It portrays a picture of a child with severe aphasia, and the emotional disturbance resulting from the isolation and lack of verbal communication and reality testing, caused by damage to the receptive areas of the brain. There is a brief review at the beginning of each term summarising what has taken place, followed by a descriptive account of the therapy sessions. It is concluded by an indication of the relationship with the therapist and how this has influenced the course of therapy.

First Term

David presented a picture of an independent, isolated little boy who would have nothing to do with me unless I had some immediate use and could satisfy an instant demand. I eventually became a possession of his which he jealously guarded from the other children but which led to no further involvement within the therapy sessions. Verbal communication was extremely limited, barely beyond the limit of a three-year-old.

Content of Interviews

When I collected David for his first interview he was reading a comic. He continued to read it all the way up the stairs and for ten minutes inside the therapy room. He then began to play in the sand tray but completely ignored my presence. His play was messy: flinging the sand and toys from the sand tray all over the room; getting the paint water and making mud pies with it and then tipping it out on the table or flinging it at the walls. He then turned around and told me to clear it up and left the room with his comic.

His attitude was like this for the first week; in the second week he began to make demands on me, making me do paintings for him while he went on with his play. He wanted pictures of his favourite nurse. Christmas trees and animals such as horses and lions. With the painting of the lion I had to put a lady, a boy and a baby inside its stomach. On all these paintings

63

David asked for his name to be put very prominently in the corner before he took them out of the room.

David's play continued to be messy, occasionally he would help to clean up and this he would do thoroughly, almost obsessively making sure everything was in its proper place before leaving the room, but at other times he just left his mess.

Second Term

David's development appears in a greater ability to express himself, showing curiosity about things around him and a desire to learn about them, and an ability to give and receive affection. He is beginning to show some signs of fear and with it anxiety, not only for his own safety but for the toys.

Content of Interviews

David told me he had gone home for his holidays with his mummy and sister Anne. He showed concern for a toy elephant that had fallen out of the window and into the gutter. He asked if it might bleed, bleed in the belly, bleed in the eyes so it would not be able to see. He would not put any water out of the window in case the elephant got wet and it hurt it. David had been playing with the animals as well as with the sand this term. He sorted out the cows and the bulls he had painted, gave them a bath and asked me to dry them. He then asked the difference between them, so I showed him. He wanted to know how they did 'wee wees' and what sort of toilet they used. I said they did not use a toilet but stood up to do 'wee wees'. He thought they stood up on their hind legs but I told him they did it standing on all four legs lifting up their tails. David then looked with me at where the animals did their 'wee wees' and their 'jobbies'. He then picked up a red Indian [sic] and asked

64

about his 'wee wees'. Two weeks later we went up to the farm to see the animals. He chattered the whole time, asking me about what we saw as we went along. He talked about mummy and daddy cows, pigs and hens. Although I explained that daddy cows were bulls and baby cows were calves I don't think he understood that though they had different names they belonged to the same family. He also found it difficult to grasp that the black patches on pigs were part of the skin and not painted on.

David still enjoys messy play with sand and water. His play, however, is becoming more constructive. For instance two weeks ago he put the sand in the squeezy container and sprinkled the sand in the water, using it as soap powder for all the cars and trucks. He then painted the squeezy container lid and very shyly brought it to me as a gift. I asked him if he would like a kiss for doing such a good job and he accepted, still very shy.

Relationship with Therapist

David has been very demanding of his time with me. There has been closer contact and he now includes me in his play, resenting it if I sit out on anything. He asks for piggy backs but has only recently received any overt affection from me. He accepts frustration better and there have been fewer aggressive outbursts this term.

Individual sessions, as well as group sessions, have great diagnostic importance. At this stage of David's treatment it became clear that the severe brain damage which he showed, probably sustained at birth, had cut off communications for him to the extent that he was totally ignorant of many of the facts of life, which most children have grasped by the age of three. It was only in the intimate situation of his therapy that this could be seen. In a group situation the other children would have made fun of him and he would have retired into his shell with a grudge, and it would have been very difficult to gain his confidence again.

During the subsequent sessions a number of other problems came up. He had a fish, and he established that it was his fish, not Ronny's, not Jimmy's, not Jacky's, but his. He tried to make the fish laugh and in other ways showed that this was a new thing for him. Then the fish died and this led to ideas of death, was mummy going to die, could people die at her age? He also tried to come to terms with the idea of 'bigness'. Then he got on to Jesus. How did Jesus stay in the sky? Could he see him if he went up in an aeroplane? How do you know about Jesus? Sunday school I think was the answer to this. He had problems still with things that were alive and things that were dead.

The eighth term recordings indicate the progress he had made and also the very considerable distance he still had to go before he caught up with children of his age.

Eighth Term

David has shown a marked improvement in his awareness and learning of what goes on about him and this improvement is also shown in his play and in his general attitudes. This awareness and curiosity extends to the people he lives with in the unit and at home. He has taken up new interests such as his animal book and his stamp collection. He has improved in such activities as cooking, playing darts and asking questions. For the greater part of the term the therapy sessions have been taken up with discussing such subjects as his mother, God, his hamster, The Man from U.N.C.L.E., Dr Who *and his friend John. I tried him in a competitive situation, which previously he had been unable to accept, and he was now able to accept this and enjoy it.*

Content of Interviews

David brought along his stamp album and as we were sorting the stamps he brought up the subject of angels again.

Where is heaven?

Why can't I see heaven when I go up in an aeroplane?

When will I die?

When will my mother die and is God looking after her?

At this point I reassured David that God was looking after his mother, but the result of this was a flood of tears and a strong denial from him that she was dead. I sat him on my knee and explained very carefully that God looked after everyone whether they were alive or dead. He soon cheered up and went on asking questions.

Can you see God?

Does God know my name?

Are there houses in heaven?

Who makes people all white and how do they get wings?

Will God turn me into a devil like Roddy? (Another boy.)

Does God hear me when I swear and see me when I pull a face?

Where does the Devil live?

Will I have children when I grow up?

When will Hammy have children?

I answered these questions as best I could.

During the following weeks David continuously brought up the subject of God and his mother who was ill and unable to see him. He told me he thought she was 22 and could you die at 22? I reassured him that people did not die unless they were seriously ill and his mother only had flu like some of the other children. The day before he went home he cooked some biscuits to take for his mother and sisters.

At darts he can cope with numbers, can add up his score sometimes in his head, more often on his fingers, and he writes this up on the board.

At cooking he can look up the index for what he wants, find the page and is beginning with my help to follow a recipe. If I point to the word 'sugar' he will go to the cupboard, find the tin of sugar and bring it. I then point to the number of ounces and he picks out the weights and weighs the sugar.

Relationship with Therapist

David's verbal communication has improved and with it a feeling of a warmer and closer contact. He has spent most of the sessions sitting talking to me or wanting to play and do things with me. He has missed his mother but has had the security to express the fear of her possible death from her illness and received comfort and reassurance from me. His fears, however, didn't disappear until he went home for a holiday and saw his mother alive and well.

This detailed work was essential if this brain-damaged boy was ever to be effectually connected up with life. Similar problems are often seen in very deprived children, and not only those who have spent much of their lives in institutions. This is also true of children with some specific learning difficulties, as was seen in the case of Robert, and predictably, with autistic children.

When David left the unit he went to a school for children with partial hearing and then to an apprenticeship with a jeweller. He became a skilled craftsman and was still working with this skill 30 years later.

David's progress in the therapy situation was paralleled by his relationships with the other children. When he first came he ran round with the other children like a little puppy, enjoying running round but with virtually no communication with the other children. Then, when his communication skills improved, he was constantly quarrelling with them, because he had no idea of the give and take of ordinary play. In the third stage he played happily with the other children because he had then learned the necessary skills.

CHAPTER 6

Children in Care

Children in care are children whose families have for some reason been unable to meet the child's needs. I think it is important to put it in this way, as we need to recognise the validity of my definition of a maladjusted child, namely a child whose needs have not been met. This takes away the idea that the child is the 'identified patient' and looks for causes of the child's difficulties outside the child. This does not mean that children whose needs have not been met do not have difficulties but it indicates the causes and points the way to rehabilitation.

In the same way I am unenthusiastic about putting too many labels on children. For one thing, children can change so drastically, either through the natural processes of maturation or in response to changes in the environment. I once saw in a residential school a child who was labelled ADHD (attention deficit hyperactivity disorder). Not only was he so labelled but he had been shown on TV as a typical case of ADHD, doing outrageous things, such as sawing off the head of his teddy bear in the family sitting-room. He was nine. When I saw him in the school to which he had been sent, he talked to me very sensibly for three quarters of an hour. Well, ADHD children are said to be all right in a one-to-one situation. I saw his teacher who told me he did not know his letters and was innumerate, but was desperately keen to learn. He would work with her with full concentration for an hour learning his letters. In his responses to the other children and to the staff he was normal, in fact a very nice little boy. This illustrates very vividly the dangers of putting these labels on children without proper investigation. In this case the child was very much the 'identified patient'. This assumption having been made, there seemed to be no need to look at the family where clearly the roots of the trouble were to be found.

I learned a great deal about children in care from a little girl of five in my residential unit. She sat on a couch in my room swinging her legs and talked about her life. Her daddy had left home and she had had another daddy. She went on to describe how he had sexually abused her. He had not hurt her and had not interfered with her vagina, but the sexual practices he had carried out with her made my hair stand on end. The original daddy whom she did not know came back to the mother, but said, 'I will come back to you but will not have that little bastard in the house.' So Amy was taken into care. She had a firm conviction that some body of people was looking after her, and was looking for a new mummy and daddy for her. She had a special person of her own, Miss –, and there was another person she had met, a nice man, and he was the one who gave her this special person, and if her special person had to go away he would provide her with another special person. Very few children in care have anything like this degree of security, though I have tried on several occasions to persuade local authorities to give it to their children.

I saw a girl recently who was in care. She was eleven and had been brought to the UK for adoption from a Romanian orphanage at the age of 20 months. She was adopted but at the age of seven the adoption broke down. She was then placed in a foster home and, as the girl put it, when she had done her stint there she was put up for adoption again. This lasted less than two years. When I saw the girl she was living in a special care unit with six other children and going to a special day school. She was an attractive child and talked to me very freely. She told me that she liked one

71

of the male staff of her present home and she had a 'key worker' who was a woman and who saw her at the worker's instigation, not the child's. She had two social workers who saw her once a month, alternating. I thought that in terms of attachment and any other model, what was being provided was a long way short of her needs.

I then heard that the social workers were collecting all the information they could get about Romania, in an attempt, apparently, to rehabilitate her as a Romanian girl. I myself have instigated searches into a child's past to help them to acquire a more stable identity, but in this case I thought that to do this was extraordinary. The child had come to this country as a baby in arms, had been rejected three times under circumstances that were traumatic for the child. I thought that giving her a Romanian identity could only increase her sense of alienation, and make her think that her rejections were because she was a foreigner.

Children's Homes

Children's Homes vary enormously. One I used to visit was in a beautiful house with an even more beautiful garden. The committee members when they visited used to say how lucky the dear children were to have such a lovely place. A snag was that the house was isolated, two and a half miles from the nearest housing estate, and the children, like the beautiful house, were isolated.

A much more successful children's home was a reception home in a big city. It was in the middle of a large new housing complex, the architecture identical with its rather drab surroundings; but the children ran in and out to play with the neighbouring children with whom they went to school. They went to tea with friends in the other apartments and their friends came to tea with them.

In terms of attachment theory, and the other relevant theories, logistics plays a big part. At the children's reception home I have just mentioned, I was asked to see a boy of four and a half. The staff said he had virtually no speech. He was not toilet trained and they were not really geared to deal with children at this level, as apparently the child could not be taught these simple skills. I said some investigation should be made before the child was written off. I asked a student psychologist who was working in my unit to test the child, and I arranged with staff of the children's home to give the child individual attention in an undisturbed one-to-one situation. The logistics showed that this could only be provided for five periods of twenty minutes on each of five days a week. This period could be managed when fresh staff came on in the afternoon half an hour before the other children came back from school. It was not possible to provide one person to give this individual attention; it had to be shared by two staff members. At this point I regret to say I forgot about the problems of this child (I had a lot on my plate). I remembered about him about eleven months later and rather diffidently asked about his progress, if any. The staff said he was 'doing fine'. He was at school, doing well, and testing by the faithful psychology student showed him to be at the upper part of the average range. This was a remarkable result, especially in terms of attachment and cognitive theories. It shows that even a small amount of individual attention can make an enormous difference to a child. In the climate and the pressure of children's homes it is often extremely difficult or even impossible to provide this, but it is worth noting how very little it takes to change a child's life dramatically. There are many good children's homes but many which could not rise to this kind of challenge.

Tim

Tim came to my residential unit when he was eleven. He was a very disturbed boy with whom no children's home had been able to cope. His mother had left home some years ago and her whereabouts were unknown. The father was said to be an alcoholic and this was borne out by the vivid demonstrations Tim gave of his coming home drunk. I thought these were sick but the boys thought they were hilarious.

When Tim had been in the unit for a few weeks I received a telephone call to say that Tim's father was dead. He had been dead for three days before he had been found behind the door of his apartment. The social worker who had phoned me said she did not think this would concern Tim. The funeral was tomorrow. I said I would bring the boy myself and asked for precise directions. It was about 75 miles away.

We arrived at the mortuary chapel where the body was lying. In the chapel were a considerable number of members of the family. They had been put off by the father's drunkenness but had rallied round at his death, as families do. An aunt whom Tim had not seen for some time cuddled him during the service, and another aunt produced a whole lot of photographs showing his father as a sergeant in the eighth army during the war, and then as a musician playing in a jazz band. The aunt said he had been very good at this. All this was quite new to Tim, who saw a very different picture of his father from the one he had known. The story had a happy ending because Tim was now a member of a quite large kinship group.

Jacky – With Comments on Conduct Disorders

I have never liked the category 'conduct disorders' as a means of labelling children, although Michael Rutter (the first Chair of Child Psychiatry at the Maudsley) and his co-workers made a very good case for this category. In any case, there are several types of delinquents. Three of the main categories are:

1) The 'well-adjusted delinquent'. These children commit offences because the game is well worth the candle. They are rarely caught, and when they are, are rarely punished – after all they have only committed this offence (for which they were caught).
2) Children who get into gangs. Peer pressure often keeps them in this subculture. Some of these children are at home in that culture but some would be only too glad to get out of the gang if they could.
3) Children who through unhappy and unpredictable circumstances find no sense or meaning in life. They are impulse ridden, their actions unaffected by their possible consequences, and apparently incapable of learning by past experiences.

Jacky belonged to the first category. He was a well-built 12-year-old, an attractive boy and a very good athlete. For him the game was well worth the candle. The children always had one afternoon a week when they could go into the town and spend their pocket money. This was as good a learning experience as anything that happened in school. Jacky was obviously well able to look after himself and he was allowed to go on his own. One afternoon Jacky came back with far more goodies than his pocket money could have purchased. When asked about this Jacky said, 'Well, you see I was walking up the vennel and in front of me was an old lady, dressed in old-fashioned things, and with a long black skirt. On the ground was a purse so I picked it up and went up to the old lady and said, "Excuse me, madam, but is this your purse?" She was rather deaf and I had to say it again. She then said, "No, little boy, it is not mine but because you have been so honest it is yours to keep." ' This was a splendid story with a lot of colourful circumstantial evidence. Unfortunately for Jacky a short time before this a man had rung the unit. He was in charge of the boats let out for hire on the river. He said, 'Tell that little bastard not to come here again, he has pinched some money from the till.'

Jacky was in care in a children's home and had no known parents or other relatives. We had a number of families who offered friendship to such children, and invited them to their homes to give them a break from institutional life. Jacky had such a family. The father was a gamekeeper and they had two children, a boy and a girl, a year or two older than Jacky. They used to have Jacky for weekends at intervals and Jacky loved going there. Then one evening he came back with a few 0.22 bullets. Luckily we found them before Jacky had had time to carry out some of the interesting experiments he had in mind with them, like hitting them with a hammer to see what happened.

This presented a real dilemma for Jacky. It was against his principles to own up to anything, and in any case he was sure that if he told the family about his crime they would never have him back. The important thing from my point of view was that for the first time in his life stealing had come between him and people he liked and who had trusted him. This could in time give him a quite different idea about crime. I asked Jacky how much this friendship meant to him. He said a great deal. I then suggested that he went for one more weekend before we told them to see how much it really did matter. I took him to the place in the car. When he came back I asked him how he had got on. He said it was fab and he desperately wanted to go back. Eventually I persuaded him to confess. I phoned the family and told them about Jacky's slip, with Jacky in the room and then Jacky said sorry. This was a very important experience for Jacky. Instead of just being good fun, something he had done wrong had come between him and something that really mattered to him, namely an important relationship with other people, in this case his family of friends. I am glad to say the family did have him back.

Foster Care

An alternative to children's homes for children who can no longer be cared for in their own homes is foster care. With difficult children and a large number of children who have suffered the trauma of a break up of their family home this can be to some extent difficult; most foster parents have inadequate support for the tasks they undertake. Some time ago Nancy Hazel, with the backing of the Director of Social Work, started a scheme in Kent, which was strikingly successful and has been followed by others. I was associated with a similar scheme run by Barnardo's called the Special Families Project. In this scheme foster parents were recruited, after careful but tactful vetting, and groups of five or six families started meeting with the social worker each fortnight. Only when the group of parents had gelled to some extent were the children sent to their foster parents who continued to meet on a fortnightly basis. These foster parents were paid, not a large sum, but considerably more than would be paid normally to a foster parent. It was regarded as a job the mother could do while remaining at home and looking after her own children. This project worked very well. The families got a good deal of help from the social worker responsible for that group, and occasionally from me as consultant to the group. I attended a fair number of the fortnightly meetings, though not all, and if some serious trouble occurred, I would sometimes make a home visit to the family. But the main support for these families was the discussion with the other members of the group. The success rate for Nancy Hazel's families was something like 90 per cent and there were comparable results with the Barnardo's Special Families Project. This would not have been possible without the support system.

For children in care, in terms of attachment theory, it is extremely difficult to meet their needs. With children in my unit I thought it was possible, with a care staff strongly motivated to give the children the love and affection they craved, together with individual psychotherapy, to bridge those gaps. The individual therapy helped to unravel some of the deep-seated problems the children had, while the group therapy helped in their relationships with other children as well as giving them some skills they did not have and thereby increasing their self-confidence. And indeed the follow-up on many of these children showed that one of the most important ingredients of attachment, namely the provision of a secure base from which exploration and the formation of new and meaningful relationships, had been achieved. It is extremely difficult in a children's home to replicate these conditions for children. All too often a question in these situations illustrates this – 'Who's on tonight?'

The situation of a child in care can be desperate. One interview I had with a boy in a residential school illustrates this. I reported that the usual semi-formal interview I have with children was not possible. Very soon after we started talking about his background he said, very reasonably, he did not want to talk about it. In view of the many rejections he had experienced I respected this – the subject must have been very painful for him. It was significant that he remembered the names of the dog and cat of the people with whom he was currently fostered, but not the names of the people themselves. I reported that I thought it very important that the social worker responsible for him should visit him regularly at times known by the boy in advance while he was in the residential school, certainly until the move to his new foster parents had been effected. The discussions with the social worker should include a member of the school staff close to the boy. The boy could then talk about it, get the facts straight, and have an opportunity to express his own views about it. I reported that I had not seen a child so disoriented for a long time. 'He feels like an unwanted parcel in a game of pass the parcel and he has a horrid feeling that a great deal of it is his fault.' There is a tendency for those responsible for children in desperate situations, as this boy was, to dodge the issue and say they will 'see him when we have something fixed up' instead of when he is feeling the pain and needs to have someone to share it with, and give him the comfort of knowing that you care.

The Koluchová Twins

In terms of development, cognitive as well as physical and emotional deprived children often function well below their potential. The case of David (Chapter 5) illustrates this very well, and Clarke and Clarke give some even more striking examples, including twin boys from Czechoslovakia as it was then, as reported by Czech researcher Jarmilia Koluchová in 1972. These twins had been placed in total isolation by their stepmother and father from eighteen months to seven years of age. The parents maintained they were severely handicapped. The boys could scarcely walk and functioned as mentally handicapped children. They went to a children's home and then to an exceptionally caring foster home. By the age of eleven they were reported to be normal in all fields. They were able to complete their schooling, taking an extra three years. Clarke and Clarke use these and other examples to illustrate the great resilience of children if only the environment can be changed for the better. This has always been my own philosophy and the basis of my practice. In most cases the environment has been the family and therapy has been directed firstly to help the child to change him or herself and secondly to attempt to modify the family environment in terms of systems theory.

79

Social Workers

The problem of children in care has never been solved adequately. I have given some examples of good care but in too many cases the child falls between several stools. One of the main difficulties is in the structure of the social work department. Social workers tend to see fewer and fewer clients as they move up through the hierarchy. At one time social workers did not continue to see clients after they had been promoted to a senior job. This meant that the bulk of the work, often with difficult families, was done by the least experienced staff. There were exceptions to this. I worked with one in charge of a large county who, when he had a very difficult family, took it on himself. These exceptions were rare. One of the main hazards children faced was the absence of continuity of care. It has to be said that social workers all too often had a formidable case load. Another big problem is that they have to undertake the supervision of families deemed to be 'at risk'. In my view this important work should be undertaken by some other official not primarily involved in being the support for the family.

I have worked with social workers for many years, they have been my allies. I have the greatest respect for them and for their profession, but too often the sheer logistics of the situation mean that they are not always able to meet the needs of children. A very disturbed child may have three social workers in nine months, with gaps between appointments.

CHAPTER 7

Autistic Children

The correct diagnosis of autistic children has never been easy, and one of the major problems is that there are as yet no generally accepted criteria for this diagnosis. This may well account for the apparent increase in the number of children diagnosed as autistic over recent years. This may be because there are more autistic children, or because the diagnoses have been widened to include many children who were not previously included, or because this is now a fashionable diagnosis. When I was first working with autistic children attempts were being made to define usable criteria for this diagnosis. The first of these criteria was as follows:

Gross and sustained impairment of emotional relationships with people.

This includes the more usual aloofness and the empty clinging (so called symbiosis) also abnormal behaviour towards other people as persons, such as using them, or parts of them, impersonally. Difficulty in mixing and playing with other children is often outstanding and long lasting.

With this and other criteria the striking thing about these children is that unlike other children who have been severely deprived, and kept under conditions of near isolation, such as some of the children described by Clarke and Clarke and others, who, when they are placed in situations where they are given adequate affection and attention become 'normal' in their relationships with other people, these autistic children, however much they improve, never achieve a completely normal and warm relationship with people. This is why I and many others regard this condition as one of dysfunction of the central nervous system. These children can be helped by intensive therapy, and, as I have described in a number of cases, they often function in the structured school setting better than they ever learn to do in less structured life settings. The development of David (Chapter 5), and especially the description of his individual therapy, illustrates the gap that has to be overcome before the child, who has inevitably missed out on such a lot of normal experience of life, can function normally. David was not autistic, but was brain damaged. His damage was not like that of autistic children, and was identifiable, but it had cut him off from a great deal of normal experience. The difficulty autistic children have is, basically, an inability to interpret correctly non-verbal and verbal emotional signals from other people.

In my unit the autistic children were treated in a setting in which the other children, although very disturbed, had the potential of getting over their problems and carrying on with a normal development. I used to worry about the autistic children because they were very vulnerable and their odd behaviour and mannerisms might, I thought, lead to an intolerable amount of teasing from the other children. But to my surprise the other children were remarkably tolerant of the autistic children, and very few difficulties of the kind I had feared occurred.

Iain

Iain came to me aged eight and a half years. He was described then as very slow and babyish. Psychometric testing gave an IQ of 24. He was rigid and ponderous in reading. There was severe emotional retardation and emotionally he was said to operate at a three-to-four-year-old level, but his limitations in the emotional field were not just those of delayed development. His reaction to emotional stimuli was abnormal and fitted only with the diagnosis of autism. There was no sign of anxiety, he seemed to be almost unconscious of other children.

In the play room he seemed almost 'mad' at first, posturing oddly, rushing around, and smiling oddly. He was severely obsessional. He memorised space stories and could repeat them verbatim. He could easily be brought back to reality. He was very insistent on being listened to. In the unit he made steady progress. In the rather more structured school situation he coped remarkably well. He could concentrate on his work. He made good progress in maths and English and was co-operative when asked to do extra work. He could cope with teasing by other children and by his teacher, to whom he was warm and friendly. He could initiate jokes himself. He would join in games and other activities with the other children. This was in marked contrast to his behaviour in the group in general. In the less structured situation of the ward he became much more odd, and could not respond to teasing or show any other signs of fun. The care staff reported that he kept mainly to himself. He continued to walk about in a rather stiff-legged fashion, with his head bowed and his arms waving about in front of him, his fingers pointing to the ground. On rare occasions he became very aggressive, and if his rage was directed to one particular child it would persist over a period of an hour. He had on these occasions to be restrained by a member of the male staff, and was a handful for them.

Similar episodes had occurred at home, though recently these had been very infrequent. Iain, like all the children in the unit, had individual therapy. This in his case was not concerned with unveiling any hidden psychopathology, but

83

with providing him with a person to whom he could relate, and to help with those aspects of reality with which he did not seem to have come to terms, very much in the way David, a boy with brain damage, was helped, as described in Chapter 5.

Joe

Joe was eight when I first saw him. He was a rather awkward looking boy, and like all autistic children was withdrawn and made very little contact with adults and none with children. He was admitted to the unit and settled in fairly well. He carried on his own routine, paying little attention to what was going on, but presenting few problems. In school, again as with most of these children he fitted in with the more structured situation well, and though he made little contact with the other children, he applied himself to his work and made quite good progress.

When the time came for him to move on to another school, he presented problems. He still had his obsessional ways and there was still a good deal of rigidity in them. It was felt that he was still vulnerable to possible bullying or teasing. Eventually a place was found for him in a school like A.S. Neill's famous Summerhill, a progressive school founded on controversial principles of personal freedom and democracy. It was very good of them to take him, as he was still a very odd boy and the school was not in any way a special school. Joe flourished there. On one occasion when I was visiting the school Joe was chairing the school committee, that is a meeting of all the pupils to decide as key school rules, which the pupils were entitled to make. Joe was conducting the meeting very efficiently. This was further than I ever thought he could go.

Subsequently Joe got an outdoor job with the local authority, a job probably below his full potential but way beyond any hopes I had for him when I first saw him. He stuck at this job for many years.

Robert

Robert came to me when he was six. He was a totally withdrawn boy and he was completely deaf. Most deaf children look at people closely in order to get clues about their world, but Robert appeared entirely absorbed in a world of his own. 'Light play' was very prominent with him. He would stand by any bright object and move his head, or the object if he could, and he seemed completely absorbed in this. There was a brass door knob on the sitting-room door and on one occasion Robert received a black eye because he was indulging in his light play too close to the knob when someone opened the door.

Eventually a teacher persuaded him to come into the class. She was using the Cuisinere rods to illustrate some points in maths. Robert showed great interest in these and soon showed that he had mastered the relationships of the rods to each other and could do sums with remarkable skill. He would even lean over and correct the sums of other children. The next step was to put the rods on a piece of paper and then put alongside each rod one or more dots denoting the value of the rod, and then put alongside these the appropriate numbers in writing. In this way Robert came to grasp the fact that symbols could have meaning. From there he was taught to read, and then to lip read.

In quite a short time this little boy who had been unteachable and also virtually unreachable became a lively and attractive child who then had to learn how to play with other children. His family went abroad, but they kept in touch with me. At the age of 16, which was the last time I heard from them, he still needed special help with his schooling. It might be argued that this was not an autistic child, but when I first saw him he satisfied all the criteria.

John

John was a remarkable boy. He was very withdrawn with people and his behaviour was very odd. He would wander round looking at the ground, sometimes saying odd things and taking no notice of people. He had good speech and on psychometric testing he showed unusual ability. He was one of those people who, if you asked him on what day his birthday would fall in 2007, would think for a minute or two and then tell you, correctly. He had good mathematical ability but I think the skill with dates was probably to do with eidetic imagery, though communication with him was quite difficult, and finding out inner processes of his mind impossible. In the unit John settled well. He was friendly and co-operative with the staff, but took virtually no notice of the other children. He lived very much in a world of his own. In his individual therapy he gradually became more responsive and one day when his mother was visiting him she said to me, 'I feel I want to take him home and cuddle him.' I said to her, 'You do just that,' and she did. John was home about three months and then came back to the unit. He was not yet able to go to any other school. Later, with his mother, he began to want to sit on her knee and he showed a great interest in her breasts. I encouraged her to tolerate this as long as she could without any real discomfort.

Another of John's obsessional habits was to wander round holding two sticks. These represented the hands of a clock. He was obsessional about time. Eventually John improved to the extent that he could go to a school which had the capacity to meet his needs.

Ivy

Ivy was referred to me when she was six. At that time she was very withdrawn and made little contact with adults, including her own parents, who were very warm and loving people, and none with other children. In general in the unit she seemed to live entirely in a world of her own, but was not difficult to manage. She was quite biddable and could follow the routine, though she showed no initiative.

She had as a therapist a girl who was good with all children but outstanding with the autistic children, with whom her patience seemed endless. When Ivy started her individual sessions she would not do anything, and would not pay attention to anything, and showed little or no interest in the therapist. So the therapist tried 'parallel play'. This involved the therapist copying whatever the child did, even if it were something like banging on a dish. For a time there was no response, and then the child seemed to resent the therapist copying her and so she took the therapist's things away. This led to considerable interaction. When the child seemed sulky the therapist would cuddle her and sing a little song, 'Coulter's Candy'. One day when the therapist was feeling particularly frustrated she sat down, put her head in her hands and pretended to have a sulk. To her surprise Ivy went up to her, tapped her on the shoulder and started to sing 'Coulter's Candy'. The child began to show great affection to the therapist and we had great hopes for her, but unfortunately she showed no improvement on the cognitive side, perhaps the ability was not there anyway. But this was one of our great disappointments. None of the other autistic children did so well on the affective side but Ivy never progressed on the cognitive side.

We were hopeful that the really warm relationship she had with her therapist, unlike that of the majority of the autistic children, would in the end lead to further cognitive development. Cognitive development is closely related to the child's relationship with people. This is well illustrated by the stories of some of the other children and especially that of Simon (Chapter 1).

CHAPTER 8

The Use of Drugs with Children

There are two main uses of drugs with children. The first
is the use of the appropriate medication for specific diseases.
Of these their use in epilepsy is an obvious example. This
is fairly straightforward, but it must be remembered that
children may have an idiosyncratic reaction to certain drugs,
as may adults, and it may be necessary to use trial and error
to find the best drug, or a combination of drugs for a particular
child. It must be remembered also that children go to school,
and that different drugs have different effects in slowing
down mental activity. I always did reaction times on the
children. It is best to wait a few days before carrying out
tests, because children who show initially quite a marked
reaction to the drug may well develop a considerable tolerance
to it. One boy I saw who had the 'grand mal' type of epilepsy
showed a definite slowing of his reaction time, but the first
term the drug was prescribed he went from near the bottom
of the class to the top.

Asthma and diabetes are other obvious diseases where the
long-term use of drugs is likely to be necessary. I have
written in earlier chapters about the psychological symptoms,
which so often accompany diseases like epilepsy and asthma.

Apart from the drugs used to alleviate the everyday diseases
of children, there is another group, which is used to try to
control difficult behaviour in children. Of these methylphenidate (Ritalin) is the most commonly used. I never used
Ritalin in the treatment of children. I never found children

– and I had some of the most difficult children anyone could find – who could not be controlled by patient use of learning theory and by the practice of a great deal of affection. I have already mentioned the boy who was supposed to be a severe and typical case but in a residential school showed no signs of this disorder himself. I think ADHD is an established condition, and in the absence of skilled treatment such as I was able to offer methylphenidate may well be of value.

As a temporary measure for really hectic children I have used haloperidol. I have when I have done this made it quite clear to the staff that this is not a treatment for the condition, it is merely a way of reducing the child's activity temporarily until they could get close enough to the child to treat them effectively.

It is in fact very difficult to determine accurately the effect of drugs on children. This was well illustrated the drug trial on the effects of haloperidol on a group of children, and especially the subsequent studies by Morris Cunningham (the psychologist of the unit) on the reliability of the nurses' notes on which the trial was based. I thought the trial did stand up and the results were valid, but Morris Cunningham's findings showed that there were many areas of doubt in these recordings. The traits on which there was satisfactory agreement and adequate spread of scores were practically all clear descriptions of obvious and frequently occurring types of behaviour, such as quarrelsome activity, teasing, anger and so on. Where these activities referred to interaction with other children the agreement was generally good. Where the behaviour was related to the nurses, such as physical aggression to the adults, seeking adult attention and obedience, there was only poor to moderate agreement. This was probably due to the different reactions of the children to the different nurses. We observed in the ward that a senior nurse might say to a child, 'Get ready for lunch', and after a brief pause the child would comply, while another, usually more junior nurse would say the same thing to the child, and the reply would be 'F--- off'. This kind of differing response to different staff members was noted in my earlier account of the end-of-term summaries.

I have used chlorpromazine on occasion, not as a form of treatment, but as a method of quietening down a child temporarily who is so hectic as to be a burden to himself as well as to the staff.

On the whole I am not in favour of using drugs as part of the treatment of disturbed children, except as a temporary measure in order to allow the staff to get closer to the child. Often the problem is with the families. I have already described how in the case of epileptic children it was some time before the families could bring themselves to exercise the kind but reasonable discipline the child needs in order to develop in a way satisfactory to all parties. I have described some of the difficulties of deciding on the effect of drugs on children in a controlled setting with skilled and sophisticated staff. The problems of making similar assessments in any other setting are obviously much greater. My own view is that children are so vulnerable, and they react so dramatically to even small changes in their environment, that I do not think there is quite the exciting future in psychopharmacology that some have advocated.

Children and the Law

In general the law is a very blunt instrument when it tries to act in a way that is in the interests of children. This applies to judicial proceedings against children who have committed offences, cases involving custody, divorce proceedings and any other legal matters where children's interests have to be taken into account. This is not to say that the lawyers are uncaring people, in fact the reverse is often the case, but the child's interest cannot always come first when considering legal matters, and all too often when there is a dispute involving two or more parents or parent substitutes, the children become pawns in the game, sometimes a rather dirty one.

One provision, which in my opinion went a long way towards meeting children's needs, was the 1968 Social Work Act of Scotland. This set up children's panels for dealing with the majority of children's problems. The panels had hearings before a tribunal of panel members, one of whom was the chairperson. Cases were referred to the hearings by the reporter, who has a similar function to the procurator fiscal, but who had additional powers and responsibilities. The fiscal responsibility was to determine whether the case was strong enough to bring to court. The reporter had much more discretion, and could see the people involved with the idea of helping them to resolve the problem themselves. Children had several important rights. One of these was to deny the grounds for the hearing. In this case the hearing could not take place, unless the reporter then referred the case to the sheriff. He then had to decide whether, on grounds of probability, the case for bringing the hearing had been made. It would be difficult to establish a comparable system in England because there is no equivalent to the sheriff. As I have said, at their best, in a hearing children as well as the relevant adults could be heard. The panels had considerable powers. They could send a child to residential school, or make an order saying that the child should reside in such and such a place, like a foster family.

Residential Schools

When I left the Royal Hospital for Sick Children in 1980 I worked for a year doing staff development and training for the residential schools in the west of Scotland. The residential schools were good, bad and indifferent, on the whole more were good. One of the best I used to visit had some pupils living in the school and attending school on the premises, others coming as day pupils, and others living in the school and going out to a local school. They also ran groups for parents, providing transport to bring them to the school. I organised three sets of courses. One, an induction course, was for staff recently joined; another was for senior staff members, while a third was called the Middle Management Course and was for staff hoping for promotion to senior posts. I learned a lot from this. One staff member was off work with flu. When he came back he told me he had sat at the window of his house watching the pre-school children playing in the street. He noticed that these little ones had better problem solving skills, and skills for getting on with people, than had the adolescents in the school in which he worked.

At one school the guidance teacher had arranged that each pupil had one half hour a week to talk to his or her class teacher on his or her own. This guidance teacher had also organised a talk by an I.C.I. senior member of staff. I.C.I. was the biggest employer in the area. He asked the children to write out an application for a job with him. Two days later he reappeared with a pile of papers. He looked through these and put about two-thirds into the waste paper basket. He then talked about some of the others, and finally interviewed about six children as though they were up for a job. To the others he said, 'Your applications were not good enough to get you on to the short list, but if you go to your class teacher with them he will help you.'

Some schools had secure units. One I visited had a unit which was locked, and each room for the boys was locked, but because the rooms were locked the boys had on display more of their possessions than I had seen on display in any school, public or private. The boys were divided into units of six, each with its own staff. Each unit had a meeting, boys and staff, every day after lunch. Here a great many problems were discussed.

The first one was about a boy who had banged on the radiator during the night. Eventually the culprit owned up. The other boys got on to him, and pointed out that they did not do that kind of thing there – it made life uncomfortable for everyone. Then there was a boy who was going home. He said he was just going to sit around and not do anything. Again the peer group got on to him. They said he was privileged to get home for a weekend and they hoped to do this as well, but if he did nothing positive about his weekend they might not get one. A third boy was being transferred to an 'open' school. He said he would go drinking, he knew how. Once more the peer group came down on him. They said this was the first time anyone had been transferred and if he ballsed it up none of them would get a chance.

The provisions for the rehabilitation of young people vary enormously. I have described some of the better provisions. It is not just staff shortages which are the problem, it is often lack of imagination.

Many of the residential schools have been closed down. I am very much against bad schools, but the closures have, I think, gone too far. There are now many more young people in secure units than used to be the case. It is rather the same with the closing of so many wards in psychiatric hospitals. Many more schizophrenic people now sleep in cardboard boxes than used to do so.

Part 2

Edinburgh

CHAPTER 9

After a number of years, I moved to Edinburgh to the Royal Hospital for Sick Children. I was very happy at Ladyfield but the 1968 Social Work Act (Scotland) had just come into force and instituted the Children's Panels and I wanted to be in on the action. In fact I did become heavily involved with the panels, as I will describe. The work at the hospital was very different from Ladyfield. There I had spent most of my time in the residential unit. I did have out-patient clinics, in the local hospital, in a primary school in Castle Douglas and at Stranraer, 60 miles away. I also visited residential establishments from which some of the children came. I also did home visits, sometimes with the social worker, though he or she did most of this work.

Edinburgh was very different. There was a small residential unit shared by three consultants but most of the work was in out-patient consultations and treatment. I inherited from my predecessor a commitment to certain schools and children's homes. I enjoyed this work and expanded it very considerably. This often involved going to one of these places in the evening when the other work was finished. I was a senior lecturer at the university and had a good deal of teaching to do. I was not too keen on lecturing but very much enjoyed seminar sessions with those in training. The schools I visited regularly included Lady Mary School in Edinburgh. This was an outstanding school, with very high standards of care and very good teaching. It was run by the organisation of the Good Shepherd and administered by a combination of nuns and lay people. Another asset the school had was a good and continuous contact with the parents. Another school was Harmeny, on the edge of Edinburgh. This was run by the Save the Children Fund, and was comparable with Lady Mary. Another was run by Barnardo's and was in Peebles. It was also a very good school. I visited these schools at regular intervals. There were some children's homes I visited regularly and others I went to on demand. I enjoyed this work and was able to make a real contribution. I had, after all, dealt over a number of years with very disturbed children in a residential setting. I enjoyed working in places where the staff were competent and where I could remain in an advisory capacity without the ultimate responsibility.

I will now talk about some of the children and their families whom I saw initially as out-patients at the hospital.

Adele

I have not seen many children who were clinically depressed. I have seen a large number of children who were very unhappy, and some who remained unhappy over a considerable period of time. Certain psychoanalytical schools have claimed that children go through depressive phases, but I think genuine clinical depression is uncommon in children, though it certainly does exist.

I saw one child, Adele, aged nine, who was depressed. Her parents were both professional people, and Adele was doing well at school, usually at top of her class. Then, at the beginning of a school term she refused to go to school and became morbidly depressed. She was sure that she had done some great evil, and would be punished for it. In fact she wanted to be punished, probably by death. If her parents took her on some special expedition to cheer her up she would say that they recognised the fact that this was probably the last time she would be able to have such an experience. Her appetite was poor but her sleep was not too severely disturbed.

I saw her as an out-patient, and prescribed antidepressant medication. This produced a marked improvement in her way of functioning and she was able to go back to school. Her mood also improved but the underlying depression remained. She still came top of her class in spite of missing two weeks at the beginning of the term.

After three months I said I would see the family in a month's time, but I warned the parents that the recovery stage of a depression was often accompanied by a period of violent hostility directed towards those nearest and dearest to the depressed person. When I next saw the parents they told me that this had indeed happened, and living through it had been hell for both of them. They told me that if I had not warned them that this could be a natural part of the recovery process they did not think they could have survived this extremely unpleasant episode. All this time the child functioned normally at school and with her friends, but gave her parents hell. This was very distressing for them as they could not help wondering what they were doing wrong. After a further month or so all this settled down and they carried on as a united though somewhat bruised family.

Jeremy

I first saw Jeremy at the Royal Hospital for Sick Children. He was in the residential unit. He was eight and the child of a single parent mother. It was usual, almost invariable, in that unit, for the children to go home each weekend to their families. Jeremy's mother always promised to come for him, but more often than not she failed to come, and left no message. Jeremy had been got ready to go home by the staff and when the mother did not appear he would blame the staff for keeping his mother from him. He would often be quite violent with them. On the odd occasions when the mother did come she would make a great fuss of Jeremy so

that he thought she was the best mother in the world. It took a long time for him to realise that it was his mother who was letting him down and not the staff. When it was quite clear, even to Jeremy and his mother, that she could not look after him he went to a children's home.

He was fortunate when he went there to have a very competent and caring care worker. After a few months the mother agreed that Jeremy should go to foster parents for a time with a view to being adopted. The foster home he went to was one of the 'Special Families' projects run by Barnado's. It was based on the pioneering work of Nancy Hazel in Kent, as detailed earlier in the book.

Jeremy's foster parents had children of their own, a little older than Jeremy. He settled well at first but after a few weeks began to be very difficult. His anger at the rejection by his mother was turned against his substitute mother, as it so often is, a pattern described John Bowlby in his work on separation and loss. Much of Jeremy's aggression was physical and it was quite hard to take. The support of the parent group was vital at this stage. As much as anything it was important for the substitute mother to be able to express her own anger and frustration at being so much abused when she was offering love and care at considerable cost to herself. Ailsa, the social worker, kept in touch and this helped to give some semblance continuity to Jeremy's life. Jeremy then settled down and was able to show love and affection to his foster mother. A disturbing episode occurred one Christmas when Jeremy took off and went to his mother's. He stayed two days and then returned of his own accord. This was when he finally decided that home with his mother was not for him.

After three years an adoptive family was found. Jeremy was able to keep in touch with both Ailsa and the foster parents, which was of great importance to him.

This is a remarkable story, with a happy ending, not

achieved without a great deal of care and love and a good deal of pain. I have seen many children who have had three or more foster homes and three or more children's homes. Not surprisingly they are then almost impossible to place anywhere. I have often wished there were more foster homes run with the imagination and the built-in support of the Barnardo's scheme.

Much of work with families is done on an out-patient basis. Family therapy is virtually always done in this way. I often did this with a co-worker, usually of another discipline.

In the field of out-patients there are infinite variations. One woman came to me because her bright teenage daughter was refusing to attend school. The husband was a very handsome, charismatic man, a university lecturer. The mother was also an intelligent woman but her self-esteem was very limited. We talked and she was encouraged and it became apparent that she and not the charismatic husband was the moving force in the family. The woman acquired a much greater level of self-confidence and in terms of systems theory the dynamics of the family changed. The girl attended school regularly.

Another family presented a pattern all too common. The mother's first marriage had ended in divorce and she married a man who had been a friend of her first husband, and in the same service. There was enormous bitterness on the part of the first husband. The boy, aged seven, spent regular weekends with his real father. When I saw the boy I was really worried about him. To any question I put to him he thought for a minute or so then looked at me again to try to see what the answer should be. He was wary in a most unchildlike way. He had obviously been cross-examined each

time he went to his father's, and often what he said did not
go down well. If he had had a good time in one place this
was not approved of in the other place. Eventually the real
father brought yet another court case demanding more access
to the boy and other demands. The father's solicitor had
carefully selected a judge who was said to be a misogynist.
I wrote a long report describing the boy's anxieties and
suggested that if the conflict continued the boy's health could
be seriously damaged. Up till then the real father had had
all his own way in the court cases but this time all my
recommendations were accepted, and I think people did at
last come to realise the harm that had been done and the
further harm that could come in the future. It was time to
stop using the child as a pawn in the game.

A Gangland Girl

One of the features of Edinburgh while we were there was
the gangs. At one time this was quite frightening, but the
police dealt with it very well. When the gangs got going it
was just like a replay of *West Side Story*. The gangs went
about in groups of between ten and thirty or more. If they
met a rival gang and the group was smaller than theirs they
beat them up. If the groups were reasonably well matched
there would be a fight, sometimes of quite frightening
proportions. The police dealt with this by putting as many
police on the streets as possible. Then when they met a
group of more than about five they became quite tough,
saying, 'Come on, break it up', and they made them disperse.
This was surprisingly effective and kept the gangs within
limits, which could be coped with.

I did not have much to do with the gangs but I had
occasional glimpses of their activity. One very pretty girl
was referred to me as an out-patient. Her family was

fragmented. Her father had left home and was working in a managerial post in England. Her mother was quite a disturbed woman, but she seemed to know most of the seniors of the social work department on Christian name terms, so it was not easy to deal with her. She kept talking about this person and that person when she really needed help rather than 'acquaintances'. The girl told me she was the girlfriend of Billy, the leader of one of the gangs, I can't remember if it was the Young Mental Drylaw or the Jungle gang or some other. She told me that once recently a group of Billy's gang, with Billy, met a boy from another gang. They beat him up, not too badly, but then one of the gang broke a bottle, gave it to Billy and said, 'There, you're the leader, you put that bottle in his face or you're not the leader.' I don't remember the outcome of this. The girl landed up in a residential school for delinquent girls. I lost touch with her but about two years later I drew up at a petrol station to fill up. The girl who served me said, 'You don't remember me, do you?' I had to say this was true. She was the girl who had been Billy's girlfriend. She told me that the residential school had scared her. There she met girls who were much tougher than she was, and much more violent. So she had mended her ways. Her mother was dead and she had not heard from her father for some time. She was engaged to a very nice boy and they were going to get married in three months' time. I told her I had not recognised her because she was much prettier than when I had seen her and I wished her every happiness and good fortune.

Colin

I also visited some of the Scottish 'List D' schools. These were for children who had committed offences and had been sent there by the courts or by the children's panels. I was asked to go to one school to attend an assessment meeting of a boy I had see as an out-patient at the hospital. At the meeting most of the staff were present. After some discussion the boy, Colin, was brought in. The staff talked to the boy, but their tone was so patronising that I felt uncomfortable. I was asked to contribute. I was not too keen to be part of such a discussion. I asked Colin if he remembered me. He said he did. I then said to him, 'Look round the people here and tell me how many you think you can con.' He looked round the room and then said to me, 'About two thirds.' The meeting took a rather different turn. The head, whom I respected, wrote to me afterwards thanking me for coming. He said, 'I think we met Colin for the first time that afternoon.'

Colin did not let the grass grow under his feet. He got hold of a copy of the relevant Act, looked it up and found that a child sent away from home under the Act could call a meeting of the children's panel and ask for review of his case. Colin did this and at the children's panel made out such a good case that he was allowed to go home. He had a good and stable home and I hoped he had learned his lesson and wished him luck.

The next three children I saw in Lady Mary School. As I have said, the school was exceptional. The standard of care was outstanding, and that of teaching comparable. The school was of primary school level and though it was a Roman Catholic School children of all faiths were admitted. I formed a very close relationship with the school. My main contact was the head, but I had links with all members of staff, and they with me. I went once a fortnight but more frequently if needed and there were frequent telephone conversations.

Edith

Edith was the third of three sisters. Her father was a professional man and there had been no problems with the family until the mother developed a severe depression soon after Edith first went to school. It is common in cases of severe depression for the sufferer to feel antipathy sometimes amounting to hatred towards a member of the family close to them, usually the husband or wife, and relationships usually return to normal when the depression is relieved. In this case, rather unusually I think, the whole of the mother's anger was directed towards Edith. When I saw Edith she had been sent to a residential school. For three months before Edith went away to school her mother had not spoken to her. When the mother wanted Edith to go to bed she would point up the stairs. The father did all he could to alleviate the situation but there was no let-up in the mother's attitude or behaviour. Edith was then six.

When I talked to her, her responses were odd, not unlike those of an autistic child. She sat on a chair at an angle so that she was not looking at me. Then she turned slowly towards me in a kind of mechanical way and spoke. Her voice lacked intonation but her answers were coherent and appropriate. In school she acted like a little automaton. She caused no trouble, did her work in school, but was a source of considerable anxiety to the care staff because of her odd manner and total lack of spontaneity.

Over the next few months Edith improved slightly, though there was no change in the home situation. Then a dramatic change in Edith's behaviour took place. In place of the quiet, biddable little girl, she became a little fiend and it took all the skills of a very good care staff to cope with her. She displayed vicious aggression, both verbal and physical, but it was what seemed like violent personal animosity directed against anyone she was with that caused the staff most distress. They needed a great deal of support. They telephoned me daily and I made several unscheduled visits to the school. It is not easy, however loving and caring you are, to have your genuine love rebuffed and instead to be metaphorically kicked in the teeth. I told them that far from doing anything wrong they had got everything right, and, in John Bowlby's terms the child had to express her anger to the substitute parents, which she had not dared to express to her own mother.

This behaviour went on for a little over three weeks, and Edith then quite suddenly reverted to being the amenable child she had been, but now she was lively, spontaneous and great fun, very affectionate to all members of the staff, and also to the other children. This situation continued for several years. Edith refused to go home and though her father was very distressed and did all he could, the mother's attitude did not significantly change, although a great deal was done to try to help the family situation. Edith went from the original primary school to a children's home for older children, connected with the original school.

Edith left school, got a job, married and had a family of her own. I think it was when she had her first child that she agreed to see her mother again.

Edith's development shows in an extreme form the effect in terms of attachment theory of a very severe depression in the mother. It is possible that initially good and secure bonding did take place between Edith and her mother although I do not have firm evidence of this. Without such a good early experience it is difficult to understand how Edith accomplished such a normal later development.

Cynthia

I saw Cynthia when she was eleven. She was in a very good residential school, and was presenting no problems in the school. She was an attractive girl at the top end of the average scale on the intelligence rating. She presented at that time no problems in the school; in fact she was well liked and doing well. The problem was with the parents. Cynthia had been adopted at an early age by two professional people. They already had two daughters, the youngest about three years older than Cynthia. The girls were clearly destined for a university career. Over the previous three years Cynthia had presented an increasingly difficult problem to her adoptive parents. I never discovered why this should have happened. The parents dealt with this problem by persuading the local authority to take Cynthia into a children's home and she only visited her home occasionally. She was then sent to the residential school where I saw her. Cynthia spent most of her holidays in the children's home. The staff and I were worried about this and I saw the parents. I suggested to the parents that the child was legally their child and asked what they proposed to do about it. The father broke down and wept, and they said they would make a serious attempt to reintegrate the child into the family. This they did, but after a full summer holiday at home they told Cynthia that things were not working out and there was no longer a place for her in that family.

Cynthia went back to the children's home and then to the residential school.

For the first few weeks of the term Cynthia was her usual friendly and co-operative self. Then she turned into an aggressive and wicked-tempered fiend. She attacked all members of the staff both verbally and physically. She was particularly vicious with her teacher, a strong, competent woman with a family. Cynthia had a biting tongue and used it. So devastating was Cynthia's onslaught on the teacher that she even seriously thought of giving up teaching. The staff including the teacher needed a great deal of support during this time. It was all very well to know about John Bowlby's work on separation and loss but to experience it in this form was quite another thing. Then, after four or five weeks, Cynthia returned to her usual pleasant self and she never looked back. It was perhaps fortunate for her that she was able to express her anger at her rejection in such a therapeutic and resilient atmosphere. Not a lot of places could have coped with it. Cynthia became particularly friendly with her teacher. She used to go to her house and showed her great signs of affection. It was perhaps interesting that her adoptive mother was a teacher. I was able to follow up Cynthia's progress for the next five years and she continued to flourish. This child demonstrated very vividly Bowlby's ideas of separation and loss. Cynthia had experienced, first separation, then the promise of coming back to the family, and then the final loss. I think it is possible that when Cynthia was younger her adoptive family may have given her a great deal of the affection, security and support that she needed. Otherwise it is difficult to understand how she survived the trauma of separation and then the extreme trauma of loss and yet remained such an attractive and trusting child.

Niobe

Niobe was referred to me when she was six. She was not like any other autistic, or indeed any other child I had seen. She was a small, waif-like only child of a single mother with an exotic, aristocratic sounding name. She took no notice of adults, nor of anyone else. She only used adults to help her to do what she wanted to do. She was restless, moving about a lot, but eye contact was nil. When you were with her you began to feel that you did not exist. She was quite incapable of attending any ordinary school. She had an amazing capacity for making three dimensional models. She liked to do this using brown or any other coloured paper and Sellotape.

I suggested she went to Lady Mary School in Edinburgh. When I went to visit after Niobe's admission I was clearly unpopular, though normally I got on very well with the staff. They said, 'Why did you do this to us? We cannot cope with this child.' I said that in four weeks' time if I suggested moving the child somewhere else they would lynch me. And so it turned out. Niobe became an enchanting and exciting child. She was still very odd, but she related more and more to those she knew, and to them she was a delight to be with.

Then the school closed down, and the education authority sent Niobe to a school in Cumbria. I was very worried about this, and wondered if any other school could cope with this strange child, and whether another school would give her the great affection as well as tolerance she needed in order to function in as normal a way as she did. I had some videos of Niobe, one taken near the beginning of her stay at Lady Mary School, and another when she had been in the school for some time, and which I had taken when I showed the child to a professional audience at the Royal Hospital for Sick Children where I worked. I showed her on closed circuit television while she played with a member of the school staff in another room. The contrast between the two videos was striking. I showed them to the new school. To my surprise they did very well for her.

When Niobe became adolescent she moved to the Rudolf Steiner School, Camphill, near Aberdeen. I visited her there.

She was then a slim and attractive girl of 13. The very good reports from the school said that in the structured setting of school lessons she was mostly well controlled. There was a very marked discrepancy between her visual perception and her auditory perception. Her visual skills were remarkable. She could draw well and with accuracy. She could also do watercolour well, putting on the paint with firm strokes, and producing an attractive picture. The other children admired her work and she would do pictures for them. She became

109

a reasonably integrated member of the class but she made no friends. A pleasant girl sat next to Niobe, but although the other girl clearly would have liked to be friends, Niobe would spend her break times on her own, often watching the younger children at play. She loved to tease other children, but if they teased her she would become upset and frequently aggressive. She could read quite well but was very poor in number work. She came to recognise notes and coins but had no real idea of the use or value of money. She could read the time on her digital watch, but the idea of time had little meaning for her. If she did anything wrong and had to be reprimanded she became very upset and sometimes aggressive. She was interested in clothes, could make or alter her own and use an electric sewing machine. She readily developed obsessions about certain things, and pursued them. She showed an almost morbid interest in some severely handicapped people, and tried to help them, but this was not apparently a genuine compassion – she seemed to want to make them perfect again, and this was not possible.

The staff noted that while much of the time she was involved in her own fantasies, and that so many of her interests became obsessions, there were times when another, much more attractive side of her nature became apparent, and she seemed to want to give and receive affection.

Niobe was a fascinating girl. She was clearly autistic, but had many talents, of which the artistic ones were the most prominent and in many ways the most exciting, but she had little ability to use these talents to improve her relationships with other people. I was sure that there was dysfunction of the central nervous system, the wide discrepancies between what she could do and what she could not do were evidence of this. And the gross and sustained impairment of emotional relationships with people remained. As an autistic child she did very well, but the severe limitations in her development remained. She was an enchanting but baffling child. Her

110

well-being was obtained at considerable cost but also with considerable satisfaction, by the care and love of a number of people.

I have mentioned some of the schools I visited. There were also several children's homes I visited, some on a regular basis, others on demand. Two outstanding ones were run by the local authority, and one was a reception home. This was situated in the middle of a housing scheme and in appearance just like all the other apartments. The children ran in and out just like all the other children living on the estate, with whom they went to school. They went to tea with their friends and their friends came to tea with them. I have already talked about one little boy who was there in the previous section 'Children in Care' (Chapter 6). Another child who was there and did very well was Vera, described below. Another very good home was run by Barnardo's. Situated in a village, the man in charge made a point of making friends with the other villagers, the result being that the children living with him went in and out of their friends' houses and their friends came to see them and have meals with them. This was the home to which Donald – discussed in Chapter 1 – went to live, and he did very well there. I also visited this home on a regular basis.

Vera

Vera was referred to me because she would not go to school. She was also referred to the children's panel. They told her that if she did not go to school they would send her to a residential school. Vera did go to school but the panel still sent her to the residential school, which I did not understand – they were usually very fair. Not surprisingly Vera did not

111

take this well. She absconded, danced on the roof, and generally caused mayhem. At the same time she began to build up a good relationship with the head teacher, who was wise and fair. The head teacher visited the home, and began to see some of the causes of Vera's problems. The parents were at loggerheads but had worked out a way of expressing their dislike of each other, and of a number of other people in a very oblique way. It was a very unhappy place to live in. The mother soon came to dislike the affection Vera had for the head teacher. She made a point of meeting the train when Vera came back after a weekend. She did not let the school know what train Vera was coming back on until the train had nearly arrived, so that the teacher had to make dash to the station to avoid letting Vera down, which was what the mother wanted.

Not long after Vera went home she came to me and asked to be taken into care. I was surprised, but less so when Vera described conditions at home. On my recommendation, and as a result of the social work department's own findings, Vera was taken into care. She went to a very good reception home, which I have mentioned previously. She settled in well. Then came the year's sports. Vera was soon seen to be a very good athlete. She was expected to win a cup for the best girl of the year. The staff of the children's home all went to watch, but Vera, being a bit of a prima-donna, did not like her place in the starting line, and would not run. After a bit her carers went home feeling frustrated, but after about three-quarters of an hour Vera appeared bearing a large cup. Everyone stared at this in amazement. After a minute or two Vera, furious, shouted, 'I bloody won it,' and apparently she had. She had done so well in the earlier heats that missing an odd race did not matter. Vera had some of her mother's skills, but luckily some nicer assets too.

Part 3

After Edinburgh Assessment Interviews and Establishing Treatment Strategies in Schools

CHAPTER 10

Altogether I had a very wide experience of a variety of residential establishments.

About the time I left the hospital the excellent Lady Mary School closed down. Two of the children were sent to a residential school privately run in Cumbria. One of these was the enchanting Niobe. I was very indignant about this; I was sure they could not meet her needs, so I arranged to go to the school. I took with me some videos I had made of Niobe. When I went to the school and saw the children I was agreeably surprised. They were managing very well including, to my surprise, Niobe. Shortly after this visit I was asked to visit the school regularly as Consultant. I agreed and went twice each term.

Assessment

The first task on going to a new school is to establish a programme of assessment. This is obviously essential before you can suggest any treatment strategies, or make any useful suggestions about the children. The details about assessment have already been recorded in Part 1 of this work but it is of such importance that it is recorded again here.

Assessment is the most important task for anyone to whom a child and his family may have come for help. Without such an evaluation, as complete as possible, no meaningful treatment strategy can be formulated, and no monitoring of the child's progress in relation to that strategy is possible.

The strategy must evolve in such a way as to meet the changing needs of the child and his or her family. There are many aspects of assessment but they all fall under three main headings:

1. **What is wrong with the child?** That is, what are his or her difficulties and what are the difficulties of those looking after and trying to teach him or her? This is the easiest part of assessment. Everyone is all too willing to tell you what is wrong with the child, usually with no reference to the other two main considerations.

2. **What is right with the child?** In other words, what are the child's assets, observable or potential? This is far by the most important part of assessment, because the assets a child has, or can be helped to develop, are all the child has to enable him or her to cope with what is wrong, and to develop in a way which will help that child to deal more effectively and more happily with their problems, and those of other people, and to get nearer to reaching his or her true potential.

3. **The child and his or her family's capacity for change.** This cannot be predicted from consideration of the first two aspects of the assessment process. Indeed these three are independent variables, and correlation between them is very low. Some children of whom I have had high hopes have not done well, while some others, against whom the dice seem to be heavily loaded, have flourished. In considering other aspects of assessment these three points should always be borne in mind.

There are other dimensions that have to be considered in relation to assessment. Four of these are: the family, education, social development, and personal attributes. They are obviously important in their own right.

1. Families are mentioned here for completeness in discussing assessment but are also dealt with in Chapter 3. One of the most important, and one of the most difficult, factors to assess is the family's capacity for change.
2. Education. Information on this point was usually reasonably accurate. There are established norms for literacy and numeracy according to a child's age. A skilled teacher will give good estimates of attention span, capacity for sustained effort, distractability, irritability and motivation.
3. Social development and skills. These are clearly important in the assessment of children but in this sphere criteria are much harder to define or determine. Because these assessments are to a large extent subjective they must be kept under constant review.
4. Personal attributes. These are closely related to social aspects, but each child is an individual in his or her own right. All children, not only disturbed ones, do not function at the same developmental level in all their activities. Parents say in frustration, 'You can do so and so, why can't you do this other thing?'

First Interview with a Child

When a child is referred to me, I read all the information available and then see the child using this form of semi-structured interview. In addition to the answers the child gives me, I record how he or she looked, how willingly they came to the interview, how they sat, the quality of eye contact, how wriggly or still the child was and what it felt like to be with the child. I also helped the staff to do these interviews themselves so that they would not be so dependent on me. Not only does this supply the school with vital information about the family not otherwise available, but it puts families in the picture, and in many cases stimulates a much greater contact with the family than had happened previously. In many cases important facts emerge from this interview of which there is no mention in the child's notes. Sometimes it is possible to have a discussion with the child about their problems, and even to indicate possible ways through them.

I regard these interviews as an essential part of the assessment process, together with discussions with the staff and information from the notes available. I always encourage Key Workers to use this format for their first contact with a child for whom they will be responsible.

Headings

1. Age   – How old are you?
   When is your birthday?
   How old would you like to be?

2. Family – Where do you live – the town, not full address?
   Who lives there with you?
   Do you have any pets – dogs, cats, etc. their names, are they special to the child?

   Father – What does he do – if unemployed, what used he to do?
   What does he like doing when he is not working?
   Does he like going out with his friends – any special night(s)?
   Do child and he do things together? What? How often?
   How do you get on with father? All right or well? Any arguments? If so, what about?

Mother – same information sought as for father.

Siblings – include not only those now living at home, but those living away, in order, eldest first. For each sibling give their age, where they live, what they do. Are they a pest, bossy or OK?

3. School – What school did you go to before you came here? What was it like, and how did you get on? What were the teachers like? Who were your friends? Were they the same friends as you had at home? If relevant, what other schools did you go to?
What is this school like? Is there anything you don't like and would change? How long do you want to stay here? If a child wants to go back to a mainstream school, would they manage? Why do they think they would manage better than they had done in the past?

4. Jobs – What do you want to do when you leave school? If you could not do that, what else would you like to do?

5. Marriage – Do you think you would like to get married one day? If not, do you think people are happy when they are married? If they say 'No' – do you think you might change your mind one day? Would you like to have children of your own? If so, how many?

6. Three Wishes – (always with primary school children, sometimes with adolescents)
If you had three wishes, as in a story, and if you could have something you wanted, or make something happen you wanted to happen, what would you wish?

1.
2.
3.

Children and young people very rarely resent this interview technique, provided the interviewer is genuinely interested in the child and treats him or her with respect, as another individual in his or her own right. Anything bordering on the patronising or authoritarian is, of course, counter-productive.

It is as well to start with something personal to the child – their age, and birthday. The question, 'How old would you like to be?' may seem a little odd, but can be illuminating. Many children in special schools (and other schools) say they would like to be 16 or 18 'because then I could leave school'. Many children say they are quite content to be the age they are. A few say they would like to be considerably younger, 'things were better then', or 'I would do things differently'.

The enquiry into the family situation helps to give you the child's perception of the situation. In cases – now quite frequent – where the family has split up, I usually ask the child if they were glad or sorry when father (or, less often, mother), left home. Most children, not surprisingly, say they are sorry. Some say 'a bit of both', and a very few that they are glad.

It will be found that this information about the family, although very simple and straightforward, rarely appears, at least in such a complete form, in the case records. All too often siblings, if mentioned, are mentioned only by name. An account, however brief, of what they are doing, and how, often gives a very fair idea of how the family is functioning.

The precise details of the father's and mother's work patterns can also be interesting. Recently I saw a child whose parents were described as stable and very caring in the records. The child told me that father worked, but in a town 30 miles from the family home, on night shift, only returning there from Friday evening to Sunday afternoon; during this period he spent his time either in the pub or sleeping. Mother worked on a checkout but at a superstore; days off Sunday, Monday, Tuesday. Her working hours were either 2–6 p.m. or 9 a.m. to 6 p.m. I asked how the boy and his 12-year-old brother managed for food. He said sometimes mother left them something to heat up; otherwise they foraged. I asked if he had a key. He said 'no', so that when mother was working they had either to stay in or stay out. I thought this was well short of my idea of a stable, caring family; and yet the only hint of this in the case records was in fact my interview with the boy.

It can be seen that, while the object of an interview of this kind is to see the world as far as is possible from the child's point of view, time and again very important aspects of the family life, its way of functioning and even a number of simple facts not previously known, emerge.

The remainder of the interview will now be seen as equally straightforward. It is interesting to note how many adolescents, as well as young children, have quite clear ideas about marriage. I always regard it as a slightly hopeful sign if a child has a definite idea of doing a job, and wants to get married and have two or more children. One boy I talked to recently said he would not get married because of AIDS; but when I asked him what he would do if he found a girl who had been tested for AIDS and found negative, he said he would marry her and have a family.

Examples of Interviews

This section describes a number of interviews with young people in accordance with the format just described. The first interview, with Steven, had a dramatic outcome and is given in narrative form. The following examples are given as transcripts, together with my comments about the interview for the benefit of the staff of the school.

Steven – Helping Children to Acquire Self-Control and Self-Management

During my first interview with Steven, he told me he was 13. He would like to be 14 as that was the age when children were allowed to smoke in the school with their parents' permission. He said smoking calmed him down when he got into an argument. He told me he lived with his mother, his two brothers, his sister and a dog. His father had left home some years ago and Steven saw him only occasionally. Steven's next younger brother was eleven, a 'pest', winding Steven up – worse than Steven, often staying off school. It was unfair that he was still at home. The younger brother was OK. He was seven. His sister was two, and was the child of the mother's current boyfriend, Bert, whom the mother had known for four or five years, and who came round at weekends. Steven thought he was preparing to move in with them but this did not worry Steven. He used to have arguments with his mother but not now. He liked his previous school but kept on getting suspended for bad behaviour and so was sent to the residential school. In this school he had ups and downs, his main trouble being constant arguments with the staff. I asked him what he would like to do when he left school. He said he would like to work with little children or to work with other people in an old people's home.

Steven had been referred to me because he was in a state of almost constant confrontation with members of the staff, especially the female staff. The same was true of the peer group, and he bullied younger children. He was at that time the most difficult and disliked boy in the school, and nobody could find a good word to say for him.

I discussed with Steven some of his obvious difficulties. He agreed with me that for some time he had been too large for his mother to control physically, and that he used this physical advantage to defy or ignore his mother's authority, leading to arguments both before and after events. I suggested to him that his way of defying female authority in the shape of his mother had a good deal to do with his attitude to the female staff in the school. He agreed that this might well be so but said that he had stopped arguing with his mother. I suggested that his mother had stopped arguing because he went his own way and she had just given up any idea of discipline for him. He denied this, but I was sure it was true and that Steven also knew it was true. I also raised with him the question of his relationship with his younger brother, suggested that his belligerent attitude to the younger boys had something to do with this. He was prepared to entertain this idea.

We then went on to discuss the idea of freedom and its relationship to inner control or self-control. I used as an analogy stories of various dogs I had known as a child. Most were ill-disciplined and had to be kept on a lead when taken for walks, while a few were well trained and could be let off the lead and had a lot more freedom and a lot more fun. I suggested to Steven that for some time he had felt pushed around by adults and sent from place to place, none of them of his choosing. I said he might well consider the idea of taking more control of his destiny, and making more of the choices himself. This would involve initially accepting more control from other people, and particularly from his mother, and choosing himself to do so. Without this adjustment, which no one could force on him, I did not see any way he and his mother could live together, and indeed it was this problem that had had a great deal to do with his coming to this school. If he accepted this it would be the beginning of his having much more say in making choices for himself and ultimately having much greater freedom.

My report on the interview said: 'Steven was quite interested in the idea of making choices for himself and becoming more involved in the running of his own life, but it is not to be supposed that one talk with me will, like a magic wand, change well-established behaviour patterns and attitudes. This will need a great deal more thought on Steven's part and a great deal of support by staff members.' I thought the technique of 'shaping' in learning theory terms might prove useful, and I went on to describe the technique. The problem with Steven was that, in the care situation, he did so little that merited approval that the behaviour modification had got into a negative phase from which there seemed no way forward. I thought shaping might reverse this negative spiral.

When I next visited the school in a month's time the head teacher asked me if I had brought my magic wand with me. I said I had no magic wand and had said so in my report. The head said that something had happened at my last visit, and the staff were now worried that Steven might be trying too hard and might not meet his own expectations, and give up trying.

It is indeed very rare for dramatic changes in attitudes and behaviour to follow one interview, but when a child's trust has been gained in counselling sessions it is almost always possible, over a number of interviews, to help child to get the idea of taking responsibility for himself or herself, and to see himself or herself as a genuinely 'growing up' person, capable of making choices, which can markedly affect his or her present circumstances and future prospects.

Charlie

Age: 13   Birthday: 24 July

Lives near Manchester with mother and one brother. They have two cats, Felix and Snowy.

Mother: Works as a secretary. Works till lunchtime on Monday, Wednesday and Friday.
Until two years ago worked full-time. She goes dancing. Dad used to be a professional dancer, tap dancing. Charlie does not like dancing.
Mother can do most forms of dancing. She also works with the amateur society. Sometimes when she is rehearsing she is out quite a bit of the evening. When this happens there is a babysitter, Jane – she has a qualification in art, and Charlie likes doing things with her. He likes doing cartoons of people and putting funny names on them. He and David and Jane did a very big one of four children, this is up on the wall in his home.

Father: Had a heart attack when he was 50, two years ago. He was professional manager of a number of shows. Charlie saw him every Sunday when he came down. In between, he was not there. Charlie was very sad when his father died. He was good fun. Charlie said he was his real father – it says in notes he was the stepfather.

Siblings: Toby, eight. A pest. He has a keyboard, a microphone, etc. and makes a horrible noise. He pesters Charlie most of the time. Sometimes he is all right.

School: In a technical college. In some ways better than West Lodge, but in other ways West Lodge is better. There was more computer time at the other school. Charlie said he gets on OK with the other boys. He still has his mates at home.

Jobs: Don't know yet. Would like to have a sports shop of his own.

Marriage: Doesn't know yet. Doesn't know about children.

Wishes: 1) To bring dad back
          2) To play for Manchester United
          3) For there to be no more wars

Charlie – notes on interview and opinion

Charlie came quite willingly to see me and talked well, adding a good deal of spontaneous comment to the answers he gave to my questions. He sat at ease in his chair and eye contact was good. He is a slight, attractive boy.

The information he gave me about his family was all new in terms of what is in his notes. In the majority of cases of children referred to a residential school, factors in the life and functioning of the family are very important in ascertaining the origins of the child's disturbance yet referring authorities rarely include this vital information in their notes. In Charlie's case the family seems to have been fragmented to a considerable degree. The father appears to have been away very much more than he was with the family, and the mother worked full-time until the father died. These are obvious problems but it is not yet clear how they affected Charlie. I am not sure whether the problems started before the father died. It would be helpful to know what Toby is like other than as a pest to Charlie.

Suggestions for treatment strategies

For Charlie. I thought Charlie was well placed in West Lodge and should do well there. Most of the time he will probably be quite biddable and work well. Given the extra help he should come near to his potential. If he does become oppositional I think this would be best handled very gently as well as firmly. Reading his story it seems that he has never learned how to come to terms with things when they do not go his own way, and so his reactions tend to be excessive and ultimately ineffective. I think he is capable of forming warm and profitable relationships with both staff and pupils.

For his mother. The mother may have a car, but in any case, works part-time and should be able to visit the school herself. As is well known, most parents by the time they have experienced the problems with the child and the child has then been 'statemented' feel guilty and to some extent hounded. It follows that in order to gain their confidence it is necessary to be seen to be on their side, and to try to see the problems from their point of view. It may be necessary to make one or more home visits in order to achieve this. Only when their confidence has been won will it be possible to make any progress in finding out how the child's difficulties have come about and only then will it be possible to help.

John

Age: 14   Birthday: 19 Jan

Lives near Manchester. Also there are mum, dad and two brothers. They have no pets.

Father: Works in a factory, day work. He likes football, watches it and plays. Watches Manchester United. He is a steward on the Manchester ground. John is not interested in football, but has been to the ground to see matches. Father also likes decorating. He goes out on Mondays and Fridays.

Mother: Works in a shop on the till, eight to four. She goes out by herself.

Siblings: Mark. Sixteen. Works in a factory. OK. Plays football. He and John do things together.
Michael. Ten. Goes to mainstream primary school.

School: Previous one in Manchester. He was thrown out for thieving. He got caught less than one in twenty times. He thinks he is somewhere between thick and bright. What does he think of West Lodge? It's better than the last school. OK. When he goes home he still goes about with mates he had before he came here (probably a delinquent bunch).

Jobs: Would like to be a mechanic.

Marriage: Perhaps at about 31.

Wishes: 1) No more violence
         2) No homeless people

John – notes on interview and opinion

John came quite cheerfully to the interview. His manner was off-hand and familiar – with a grin much of the time. Eye contact was very poor, and he was very restless, sometimes swinging round to try to see Helen, who was present at the interview, but Helen was sitting almost behind him and he did not make any contact with her. In spite of his off-hand manner and his restlessness he gave a very good interview, answering questions readily though there was little spontaneous comment.
    He presented himself as a cheerful rogue, streetwise and

well in control of his life, yet in the latter part of the interview, which attempts to get an idea of the child's aspirations and his view of the future, he spoke of serious issues in a serious way, and looked forward to doing a worthwhile job, to getting married and having a family of his own. His wishes were even more surprising. I thought they came out of him as quite genuine, as did Helen. They represented the aspirations of his intact, hard-working family rather than the cheerful rebel.

I thought this boy was in a situation possibly of rebellion against his father, possibly under peer group pressure, possibly both. I thought he was 'redeemable' but this would need skilled counselling while he is in the school. Without this I think he is capable of 'getting by' in the school, playing the system and leaving the school rather better educated but with the problems, which led to his referral to the school, basically untouched.

Suggestions for treatment strategies

If I were to undertake his counselling I would try to interest him in choices. I would suggest to him that little boys who committed indictable offences were often quite cute and were treated gently, but as they got older were less and less cute and looked more and more like a menace. He still had choices: he could continue as he was with people treating him more and more harshly as he grew older until there was no way back and he was stuck in an exciting but precarious life. The fact that he was quite good at the crimes would be likely to prolong the process but make it less and less easy to make other choices. It needs to be very clear to him that you are not attempting to pressure him in any way, but are only interested in discussing choices with him. Sometimes it is necessary to give the impression that you could not care less which choices he ultimately makes, the whole thing

129

being a matter of considerable, but mainly academic interest to you. We should never carry this attitude too far but a hint of it may turn the scales.

In normal circumstances if anyone goes to a doctor or other professional for help this is a contractual situation. This does not apply to children and their families in this situation. The child has come to the school because of various statutory procedures including 'statementing'. To attempt any therapeutic help, it is first necessary to obtain the trust of the individual you are trying to help so that you are no longer just another authority figure.

In this case nothing useful can be done without the active co-operation of the father and almost certainly the mother too. As I have said it will be necessary to get the father's trust first. Then his feelings about his son can be assessed. Both the older brother and the younger seem to be on the straight and narrow path and the father may be puzzled as to why the middle boy should be off the rails. In some cases it is necessary to 'sell' the child back to the parent. The father almost certainly has a car and with careful negotiation may well be induced to visit the school. The negotiations will be necessary as he is a busy man and probably thinks of himself as an important man. Success in such a venture would be very rewarding for both the boy and his family.

Barry

This interview was done by a member of the staff who had discussed this interviewing technique with me and who had sat in on interviews I had done with children.

Aged: 13   Birthday: 5 May 1986

Barry would like to be 20 so that he can do what he likes.

Family: Barry lives in Warrington with his adoptive mum and dad, two sisters (not adopted) and a nephew of the parents. He has a rabbit called Lucy, which is his own.

Father: An HGV driver away Monday to Friday. He enjoys doing DIY around the house at weekends. Barry and dad have been camping near Chester every weekend over the summer after dad bought a new motorbike. They get on OK, but sometimes argue about silly things.

Mother: Works as a child minder. She looks after two babies, three primary school children and sometimes Barry's two-year-old nephew. She works in a bar on Thursday and Friday nights, and goes to Bingo on Monday. Barry often goes out with mum and dad at the weekends, recently they have been to Southport Air Show. Barry gets on with mum all right but they argue about 'everything'.

Siblings: Emma. Twenty-one. Living at home and working. She has a two-year-old son called Dan who lives with the family. Dan is Barry's godson and Barry is very fond of him. Barry gets on OK with Emma.

Michaela. Seventeen. She lives at home and is doing a college course in hairdressing. Barry says she is 'not bad'.

School: Barry went to High School previous to West Lodge. He found it OK, but was sent out of class a lot. There was one particular teacher, a Mr Black, who took him for history and was his tutor, which Barry liked. He felt that Mr Black understood the problems that he was facing. Barry had a few friends at the school and also he hangs around with them in the evenings now. Barry left as his mother felt the school was not giving enough support. West Lodge has been OK so far though he does not like some of the teachers. He would like to go back to mainstream but knows his behaviour

needs to improve and he needs to catch up with his work
He thinks that if he can learn at West Lodge he will cope
better at mainstream. Although Barry would like to go back
to mainstream he could also see himself staying to do his
GCSEs at West Lodge. Barry likes being in a smaller class
and feels his needs are being met better here.

Jobs: Barry would like to be in the army when he gets older.
Alternatively he would like to work for one of the emergency
services. He thinks these would be exciting jobs.

Wishes   1) Not to have ADHD
         2) To be rich

Barry was interviewed shortly after being very disruptive.
Going through the interview had a visibly calming effect on
him. He seemed happy to talk about himself and some of
his experiences. He held reasonable eye contact throughout
and sat quietly without fidgeting. Barry was interested to
look through what I had noted down after the interview but
did not want anything reading back to him.

We discussed Barry's being adopted. He found out a few
years ago when his mum told him without any build-up or
warning. He said he ran to his bedroom and felt upset and
confused. He says he feels OK about being adopted but
sometimes uses it to upset his parents, especially mum ('you're
not my real mum'). He does not really mean it but sometimes
feels that he does. Barry has a book at home with information
about biological mum and dad with photos in it that a social
worker prepared for him when he was adopted. He says he
does not look like his real parents but actually looks quite
like his adoptive dad. Barry stated that he was adopted as
soon as we started talking about his family and enlarged on
the subject with very little prompting.

Elsie

Aged 12

Lives near Manchester with mum and brother. They used to have a rabbit but it died. She thinks a fox in the garden scared it.

Mother: Works in the house, goes shopping, sits watching TV. Has friends in. Used to go out clubbing with her friends, not any more. Elsie and mum go shopping together, mum does homework with Elsie. Gets on quite well with mum, they argue sometimes.

Siblings: Peter. Nineteen in November. Batters Elsie sometimes, gets his own way with mum. Elsie gets 30p a day. He's a bit of a pain – the biggest ever. Goes to college. Keeps losing jobs – used to lie and say he is not well. He can be nice to her.

School: Went to West Linton – it was a residential unit but she went as a day pupil. All right, some nasty kids, same here but they are stricter with them here. West Lodge is fine, only four more years. Would like to go back to mainstream 'but I can't' – then 'I don't want to go to mainstream anyway'.

Jobs: Would like to go to college. Likes maths, would like to do hairdressing, would like to live with mum, look after her, possibly have a flat as well, visit mum every day.

Wishes: 1) £100 for mum
2) Take mum to Disneyland
3) Buy a big house

Elsie thinks she is a nice person with nasty bits.

Elsie – notes on interview and opinion

When Elsie first came in and sat down she was rather hunched up, and was sucking her thumb. She soon settled down and talked well.

I thought the most striking thing in her story was her curious relationship with her mother. There is an excellent description of an interview with Elsie and her mother in Nigel's notes on his home visit. Elsie is obviously very attached to her mother (see her 'wishes' in my interview and her account of her life when she gets a job), but Elsie and her mother seem curiously the same, neither listening to the other.

I thought Elsie was basically a very nice person. I thought that if possible it would be helpful to have some more interviews with Elsie and her mother together to get them both to listen to each other. I think this curious relationship is at the root of Elsie's problems. I think she will settle well in West Lodge but unless her relationship with her mother is tackled successfully her underlying problems will not be touched. They can only be approached by seeing Elsie and her mother together. I think Elsie's violence outside the home reflects the internal conflict with her mother. She is apparently all concern for her mother, all her wishes are directed towards things for her mother, and yet Nigel's vivid description of a discussion with them both shows them both talking at once and repeatedly telling each other to shut up. It seems as though the aggression she feels towards her mother comes out in the violence and the confrontational attitude she shows towards other people. The situation is unusual, and not an easy one, but I think within the school's capacity to deal with it.

Establishing Treatment Strategies for Children, including Counselling and Supervision

All establishments that cater for children have to make themselves responsible for meeting children's needs. In the case of residential establishments the onus on them to meet a greater number of children's needs is more taxing. There are many ways of defining children's needs and the following is one simplified form.

1) The need for security.
2) The need to belong to and be accepted in a group.
3) New experiences.
4) Giving and receiving affection.
5) Identity and feelings of worth and value.
6) Independence and responsibility.

Children come into residential schools for various reasons. For a time many of these children were called 'maladjusted'. My definition of a maladjusted child is a child whose needs are not being met. This switches the 'diagnosis' from the child to the variables outside the child where it rightly belongs.

Although children cannot be held responsible for the circumstances that bring them to a residential school, if they are to achieve a state in which their behaviour is more acceptable they must ultimately accept a considerable degree of responsibility for themselves, often, if it is to be successful, responsibility that would normally be beyond their years.

In a good residential school the children find a regime that is ordered, that is predictable, and is implemented by staff who are confident of the clear guidelines by which they operate, and are caring towards the children. This regime, and the way it is operated, will go a long way towards meeting the needs listed above as 1), 2) and 3); and some way towards meeting the very important need 4). But the milieu itself, however good, has only limited capacity to meet the equally important needs 5) and 6). It is here that seeing the child individually by their key worker can be used to add to the effectiveness of the regime in meeting the other needs, and above all to involve the child in his or her own treatment. The first object of this is to help the child to accept external control, which is the first and an essential step towards internalising control, that is, acquiring self-control.

By seeing the child as an individual, giving him or her specific appointments – and keeping them, the child can be helped to develop an identity of his or her own, and a feeling of worth and value. In this context trust can be established together with real communication with the child, and they can be helped to gain a degree of independence, and to begin to take responsibility for their own actions. They can also be helped to see the value of giving up some short-term goals, aimed at immediate satisfaction, for more worthwhile long-term goals, offering more important and lasting values and achievements. In relation to these ideas and aims short cuts are ineffective, and usually counterproductive. It is of little use to say to a child newly admitted, 'Now it is all up to you.' Meaningful discussions involving the child in decision making, and accepting responsibility, come only after the establishment of trust. And there is no immediate way to trust, particularly with children who have often been let down in the past. Trust is a matter of experience, and that involves an inescapable time factor. It is very important in all your dealings with a child to be seen by them as entirely trustworthy. Children live in a more black and white world than adults, and are unfamiliar with the compromises that play such a large part in adult relationships. If you have to break an appointment with a child, tell them beforehand, make another and keep it.

Communicating with Children

Counselling is one of the important ways of finding out what children's individual needs are, and in some cases can go a considerable way towards meeting them.

The first, and indeed the main problem, is to establish communication with the child. This is not always easy, for though with some children just talking presents no difficulty, real communication, which involves an exchange of ideas, is more of a problem. In the early stages, the less you say, the better. My own children taught me about this. One daughter aged 13 said to me, crossly, 'You always find out all about us – but that's because you never ask' – that made me think.

Another aspect of children's talk, when you are first getting to know them, is that a great deal of what they say may not coincide with your own ideas of reality. This is not surprising, and it applies to adult attempts at communication. You have only to read an account of a debate in the Houses of Parliament to appreciate some of the varying aspects of reality – in many cases they might all be talking about quite different subjects, and certainly their perceptions of the same subject are widely different. Reality, in the sphere of communication, is many-hued.

1) The only actual reality is what the child actually said.
2) This may correspond with an objective reality.
3) It may correspond to reality as you see it.
4) It may correspond to reality as the child sees it.
5) It may be said deliberately to deceive you.
6) It may be fantasy in which the child more than half believes.

There are many pitfalls in a search for truth. In any case,

in the early stages of getting to know a child it is better just
to accept what the child says at face value – in fact this
may be the only way of gaining the child's confidence.
Confidence implies trust, and trust, as has already been said,
is a matter of experience. It should be said this kind of
acceptance of what a child says is acceptable, probably
essential, in the therapeutic situation of a key worker in an
individual session with a child. When that same staff member
is dealing with the child in a group situation, and the child
says something which you have good reason to believe to
be untrue, it is equally important to say to the child, 'I am
sorry, I do not think that is right, and I am going to act
accordingly.' Perhaps surprisingly this causes little confusion
or resentment in the child's mind. Mostly they have a very
good idea of what the score is.

I have talked here about a therapeutic situation. There is
much confusion about the idea of therapy, and a good deal
of nonsense has accumulated round this idea. Therapy implies
treatment, and treatment is basically trying to help someone
with a specific problem, for which you have some skills,
whether it is a sore throat or some more complex behavioural
or psychological problem. Whatever method is used, the
essence of therapy is:

1) Arriving with the person you are trying to help at a
   consensus as to what the reality of the situation is.
2) Coming to terms with that reality.
3) Deciding by consensus what you are going to do
   about it.

It is as well to remember that a great many children in
school have very little experience of real communication with
adults, in the sense that what they have to say, and what
they think, are really listened to. So that the establishment
of communication with children often requires a great deal

of patience and understanding. All too often the bulk of communication between adults and children, in families as in school, is confined to the adult saying, 'Do this' or 'Don't do that', and the child saying, 'Can I do this?' or 'Can I have money for that?' or in school to answering questions. The establishing of real communication with a child can be as exciting for the adult as it can be for the child, for whom it can open up new worlds.

Essential Tasks for Key Workers

1. To get to know thoroughly the child and his or her family background. This involves:

a) Going carefully through the file and summarising the relevant information – very much a summary. Good summaries are more difficult to write than fuller versions.
b) First and subsequent interviews with the child. I have described above a format for first interviews, which I have found useful, and given indications about how subsequent interviews might go.
c) A short summary indicating where the child is in terms of his or her educational development, social development and emotional development.
d) From the above data a brief formulation of the treatment strategy as agreed with senior staff members.

I have found this brief summary extremely helpful. It should be readily available to all staff members, and always available when the child is discussed at staff meetings.

It is part of the initial task of the key worker to know the child and his or her background thoroughly, so that not only is the child a real person to the key worker in the context of a real background, but the key worker is able to keep his or her colleagues constantly in touch with this real person.

The continuation of the initial task will involve updating the summary in terms of:

a) Developmental progress the child has achieved.
b) The staff's changing perceptions of the child and his or her family.
c) Any prescribed modifications in the treatment strategy to keep pace with the child's development.

2. After completion of the first task the ongoing relationship of the key worker with the child needs to be defined, in full discussions with the key worker's supervisor. The needs of individual children vary greatly. Some with severe disturbances may need skilled and quite long-term therapy, while for others who have already achieved a greater degree of integration, the therapeutic role of the key worker, though important, will be less intense and more of a supportive nature. The one role the key worker should not be cast in is that of the person mainly going over the child's behaviour and pointing out where he or she has gone wrong.

Suggestions for an Integrated Scheme for Staff Development

The establishment and maintenance of an effective scheme for staff development relies on two main structures, an efficient line management and an efficient communications system. The two are closely linked. The head of a school or department cannot see all members of staff all the time, and is even less able to see all the children. He or she must be available to see individual members of staff, when needed, either by them or by him or her. He or she must also see individual children when needed. But to keep in touch with events day by day, and week by week, he or she must rely on the two systems already mentioned.

140

Starting with the children, each child will have a key worker. The role of the key worker has already been discussed. The key worker will take his or her work with the child to his or her supervisor, and it will be discussed. Supervision is a mutual learning situation. I always hoped people I was 'supervising' got anything like as much out of it as I did. In the early stages the supervisor will do best by reinforcing the positive aspects of the counsellor's work. This increases confidence, much needed at first, and increasing awareness of a child's reactions can be stimulated by discreet questions. For example, if you ask about a child's eye contact, and the counsellor has not noticed this, it is obviously not helpful to register surprise, much less disapproval. The supervisor merely passes to another topic. He or she will find that when the topic comes up again due note will have been taken of this aspect of behaviour.

Supervision sessions should be a shared and enriching experience for both people taking part in them. A too didactic approach inhibits free communication. It is more helpful for the supervisor to say, 'It looks to me as though such-and-such might be what is happening, how does this strike you?' Any differing opinion from the counsellor should be given a serious hearing, and in fact encouraged. Then they can both say, 'We will see how it turns out.' All too often we are guessing when it comes to interpreting behaviour, and observations we are not sure about are a strong indication to look harder for more evidence. This process is important as an aid to sharpening perception.

I think to begin with supervision sessions should be primarily task oriented, in other words about the children. If a real trust is built up over a period of time between staff members, the inevitable tensions arising from the job will readily surface, and may well provide the supervisor with more problems than he or she can comfortably cope with.

When a staff member takes over the role of counsellor it

is important that there should be a clear-cut definition of aims, including long-term and short-term goals (these latter may be the establishing of trust and communication). Without this clear-cut definition of aims, and the need to modify them as the child develops, counselling and supervision have little meaning and can cause mainly frustration.

Another vital part of staff communication and development is in the regular staff meetings. Such meetings of senior staff with the head have already been mentioned. There will in addition be regular meetings of staff groups to discuss the children, and also administrative matters. I have found that it is helpful for staff members to take it in turn to keep minutes of these meetings. From the sheer logistics of this these minutes need to be very short, not recording the discussion, only the decisions arrived at during the meetings.

I attach great importance to the essential parts of notes being typed. I used to spend untold hours wading through case files. The average time it took me to read and annotate one file varied from 15 to 40 minutes, and I, with years of experience, was very quick at these tasks. I think the minimum that should be typed is the key worker's summaries, updated by discussions in staff meetings or with the supervisor. In one of my units in which I worked for 18 years the care staff notes were typed, the only ones in the whole hospital. Having your notes typed, and read, wonderfully concentrates the mind. Another important point is to make sure the contributions and particularly the difficulties of the less experienced staff are sufficiently valued at meetings. Often the account of a child's behaviour by a senior staff member will give a good idea of the child's potential with skilled handling, while the story from a less experienced member will give, in many cases, an idea of what the mother or father is up against.

The final link is the senior staff meetings with the head. These complete the link, providing the head with vital and detailed information about the progress of the children, and of the development of the staff. Here policies can be discussed, and ways of implementing them decided. It is here also that the senior staff members can get the support and encouragement they need.

APPENDIX

Ladyfield staff

Morris Cunningham   He got a double first in Moral Philosophy at Cambridge and then took a degree at London University. He was the psychologist to the unit and made a very great contribution to the whole tone of the unit and to its development.

Miss Sutherland   She was the original head of the care staff. She had great administrative skills and could show affection to the children. She was important in giving the unit a good start.

Alfred Gunn   He was a very erudite teacher who had an amazing rapport with children. There was a wide age range and some were very bright while some were dull. Without his exceptional skills and stamina it is doubtful if the unit would have got off the ground.

Kenneth Cameron   He was the first Consultant in Child Psychiatry at the Institute of Psychiatry in London. With him I had my first experience of child psychiatry at the Maudsley Hospital. He wrote a very helpful paper of guidelines for care staff working with children, which I found very helpful when setting up the Ladyfield Unit.

Tom Dudgeon　　He was the head of the second part of the unit, a key role.

Juliet Harper　　An occupational therapist who, while good with all children, was especially skilled with the autistic children.

There are many others who could be named, but space does not permit.

SELECT BIBLIOGRAPHY

Bowlby, John, *Attachment and Loss, Volume 1: Attachment, Volume 2: Separation – Anxiety and Anger, Volume 3: Loss – Sadness and Depression* (paperback editions, Penguin, 1991)

Cameron, Kenneth, 'A Psychiatric In-Patient Department for Children', *Journal for Mental Science*, Vol 95, 1949

Cameron, Kenneth, 'Postgraduate Training in Child Psychiatry', *American Journal of Psychiatry*, Vol 106, 1950

Clarke, Alan and Clarke, Ann, *Early Experience and the Life Path* (Jessica Kingsley, 2000)

Dockar-Drysdale, Barbara, *Therapy in Child Care* (Longman, 1968)

Eysenck, H.J., and Rachman, S.J., *The Causes and Cures of Neurosis* (Routledge & Kegan Paul, 1965)

Freud, Sigmund, Ed. James Strachey, *The Collected Papers of Sigmund Freud* (Hogarth Press, 1950)

Howells, John G., *Modern Perspectives in Child Psychiatry* (Oliver & Boyd, 1965)

Lorenz, Konrad, *On Aggression* (Methuen, 1966)

Minuchin, Salvador, *Families and Family Therapy* (Harvard University Press, 1974)

Neil, A.S., *Summerhill* (Pelican, 1968)

Piaget, Jean, *The Origin of Intelligence in the Child*, International Library of Psychology (Routledge & Kegan Paul, 1953)

Redl, Fritz and Wineman, D., *Children Who Hate* (Free Press, 1951)

Rutter, Michael, *Helping Troubled Children* (Penguin, 1977)

Satir, Virginia, *Conjoint Family Therapy* (Science and Behavior
    Books, 1967)
Winnicott, Donald W., *Playing and Reality* (Routledge, 1971